The Healthcare
Compliance
Professional's
Guide to

Policies and Procedures

Richard P. Kusserow

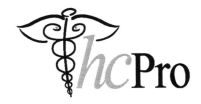

The Healthcare Compliance Professional's Guide to Policies and Procedures is published by HCPro, Inc.

Copyright © 2008 HCPro, Inc.

All rights reserved. Printed in the United States of America.   5   4   3   2   1

ISBN 978-1-60146-172-8

HCPro, Inc., provides information resources for the healthcare industry.

HCPro, Inc., is not affiliated in any way with The Joint Commission, which owns the JCAHO and Joint Commission trademarks.

Richard P. Kusserow, Author
Melissa J. Varnavas, CPC-A, Editor
Melissa Osborn, Executive Editor
Lauren McLeod, Group Publisher
Susan Darbyshire, Cover Designer
Jackie Diehl Singer, Graphic Artist
Matthew Kuhrt, Copyeditor
Lauren Rubenzahl, Proofreader
Jean St. Pierre, Director of Operations
Darren Kelly, Books Production Supervisor
Susan Darbyshire, Art Director
Claire Cloutier, Production Manager
Paul Singer, Layout Artist

Advice given is general. Readers should consult professional counsel for specific legal, ethical, or clinical questions.

Arrangements can be made for quantity discounts. For more information, contact:

HCPro, Inc.
P.O. Box 1168
Marblehead, MA 01945
Telephone: 800/650-6787 or 781/639-1872
Fax: 781/639-2982
E-mail: *customerservice@hcpro.com*

Visit HCPro, Inc., at its World Wide Web sites:
www.hcpro.com and *www.hcmarketplace.com*

2/2008
21381

Contents

Introduction

About this book

The book is designed to provide an introduction to compliance program development by addressing the building of the program's structure. To assist in this effort, this manual contains numerous templates that can be adapted to the specific needs of any organization. It addresses all seven standard elements of a compliance program outlined by the United States Sentencing Commission as elaborated on and adapted to the healthcare industry sector by the Office of Inspector General (OIG).

Templates

There are 41 templates in this manual that compliance officers can use to develop or enhance an effective compliance program. In addition, there are a variety of practices, guidance, and suggestions for the efficient and effective management of a compliance hotline program. The templates can be tailored to the specific needs of any organization. Take time to ensure that the documents adopted by your organization fit your organization's culture.

Best-practice tips

This manual includes a number of best-practice tips to draw attention to standards that will enhance and improve compliance program development, operation, and effectiveness. A number of citations are provided for those who would like to find original government source documents on the subject.

Cross referencing to OIG Compliance Guidance

The original OIG Compliance Guidance is appended to this manual as *Appendix I* located on the CD-ROM. It cross-references to templates provided in the manual for easy verification that all the material elements called for in an effective compliance program have been addressed. The reader may wish to peruse this appendix first and then work through the manual, continually referring back to this source document.

This manual is organized as follows:

Chapter 1: Background and overview

This section addresses the objectives of this manual and how it can be best used. It includes the background, framework, and context for compliance programs through the examination of various legal, regulatory, and standard-setting guidelines provided to organizations in the healthcare industry.

Chapter 2: The seven elements of a compliance program

This section addresses the seven standard elements of a compliance program used by the United States Sentencing Commission and the Department of Health and Human Services (HHS) OIG, along with 41 template policies, procedures, and other documents that can be used in building the structure for the program at your facility.

Chapter 3: Monitoring, communicating, and responding to government agencies
This section addresses communication from and to the Center for Medicare & Medicaid Services (CMS) and the OIG

Chapter 4: Compliance program implementation planning
This section focuses on suggested compliance implementation strategies utilizing the templates and tools included in this manual. It reduces the process to four major steps, with descriptions and directions for each. It includes a template for objective-setting, defining tasks, and statements of deliverables for each task for the four steps.

This can be used as a starting point for a plan under development, or it can be modified depending on what tasks and deliverables might already have been addressed. A second template outlines a suggested timeframe for completion of the 21 tasks identified.

Disclaimer

This publication is designed to provide accurate, comprehensive, and authoritative information on the subject matter covered. However, the publisher and author do not warrant that the information contained herein is either complete or accurate. This manual is published with the understanding that neither the publisher nor the author is engaged in rendering legal or other professional services. If legal advice or other expert assistance is required, the services of a competent professional should be sought to address the specific issues or concerns.

About the author

Richard P. Kusserow is the founder and CEO of Strategic Management Systems, Inc. In that capacity, he leads the evaluation of difficult compliance issues. He began developing, evaluating, and enhancing compliance programs in 1992. He previously served for 11 years as the Inspector General (IG) of the HHS, where he was responsible for all investigations, audits, and inspections performed on behalf of the department.

In addition, Mr. Kusserow worked with the FBI for 11 years prior to accepting a presidential appointment to IG. He was twice elected as national president of the Association of Federal Investigators and once as national president of the Association of Government Accountants. He was appointed by President George H. W. Bush to the National Law Enforcement Commission and by the attorney general to the Economic Crime Council. He served on the President's Counsel on Integrity and Efficiency (PCIE), President's Counsel on Management Improvement (PCMI), and Chief Financial Officers Counsel.

Mr. Kusserow is a frequent speaker at conferences and events, and he is often called on for media interviews on federal policy issues. He has published dozens of journal articles and is the author of several books, including:

- *Management principles for asset protection* (1995), Wiley and Sons (1986)

- *Corporate compliance policies and procedures: Guide to assessment and development* (2000), Opus Communications (HCPro, Inc.)

- *Corporate compliance education & training programs: A manual and guide* (2001), Opus Communications (HCPro, Inc.)

- *Sarbanes-Oxley: Best practices for private and nonprofit health care entities*, AIS (2003)

- *49 Steps to Implement Sarbanes-Oxley Best Practices*, AIS (2006)

- *Ultimate Hotline Manual: Tool Kit & Practical Guide for Establishing/Managing a Hotline Operation*, NHS (2005)

About Strategic Management

Strategic Management was founded in 1992 by Richard Kusserow, former Inspector General of HHS. Over the past two decades, Strategic Management has provided regulatory analysis and compliance program development, implementation, evaluation, and review services to the healthcare industry. The firm possesses unique expertise involving healthcare laws and regulations, such as the Anti-Kickback Statute, qui tam actions, Safe Harbor Regulations, Health Insurance Portability and Accountability Act (HIPAA), Medicare/Medicaid regulations, Sarbanes-Oxley compliance, and others. Strategic Management has a strong track record in providing valuable management strategies for dealing with difficult regulatory and enforcement problems. It is headquartered in the Washington, D.C. suburb of Alexandria, VA.

The firm's principals have worked day to day with the executive, enforcement, and regulatory agencies of the federal government, as well as with Congress, the Office of Management and Budget, and the top health, defense, and labor policy officials within the administration. Strategic Management pioneered healthcare compliance program development and has assisted more than 600 organizations and entities with compliance program services.

Strategic Management also offers an array of services and support, fair-market-value determinations, evaluations of arrangements, compliance education and training, policy and procedure development, tailored work plans, and guided implementation. A variety of organization types, such as national health systems, regional health systems, small hospitals, laboratories, teaching facilities, medical schools, insurance companies, and long-term care facilities, have benefited from Strategic Management's compliance experience and knowledge.

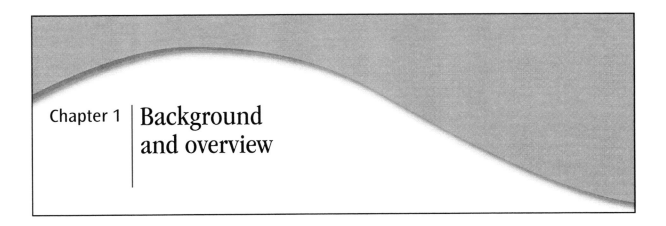

Chapter 1 | Background and overview

Compliance program structure

Building an "effective" compliance program does not end simply with the implementation of the foundation, or plan, for its operation and management. This book includes more than three dozen templates related to making a compliance program operate the way it should, including:

- Compliance office relations with legal counsel, finance, and human resource management (HRM)

- Compliance investigations and management

- Reporting of findings and resolution of issues

- How to deal with subpoenas and search warrants

- Requesting advice from government agencies

- Gifts, entertainment, discounts, promotions, and business courtesies

- Workplace safety issues

- Conflicts of interest, nepotism, and outside employment

- Protection of documents and other assets

- Enforcement

- Confidentiality and non-disclosure agreements

- Table of penalties for compliance infractions

- Compliance program reviews

In 1997, the Office of Inspector General (OIG) began compliance guidance for various sectors of the healthcare industry. All of the guidance documents stress that every compliance program should require the development and distribution of written compliance policies that promote a commitment to compliance.

The OIG compliance guidance is not mandated by law or regulation but is rather "suggested." The OIG notes that its guidance promotes voluntarily developed and implemented compliance programs for the healthcare industry. It is intended to assist in the development of effective internal controls that promote adherence to applicable federal and state law and to the program requirements of federal, state, and private health plans. They note that the adoption and implementation of voluntary compliance programs significantly advance the prevention of fraud, abuse, and waste, while furthering the fundamental mission to provide quality care to patients.

In developing a compliance program, compliance policies fall into two general categories:

- Those that relate to the operation of the compliance program

- Those that relate to specific areas of compliance risk

In the former, the compliance officer bears the responsibility for the development, implementation, management, and enforcement of the policies, as well as the adherence to the specific procedures related to those policies. In the latter, the development, implementation, management, and enforcement of the policies fall on the operations managers responsible for the risk area, with oversight by the compliance officer. In both cases, the policies should be developed under the direction and supervision of the compliance officer and the compliance committee. Once developed, the policies should be disseminated to all individuals affected by the particular policy at issue, and appropriate training and monitoring should be conducted.

This manual is designed to assist in providing an elemental structure for a compliance program. It focuses on the basic policies related to the operation and management of the compliance office referenced by the OIG in its guidance documents. This approach to the basics is consistent with the stated intent of the OIG in its *Compliance Guidance for Hospitals*, wherein it states,

While this document presents basic procedural and structural guidance for designing a compliance program, it is not in itself a compliance program. Rather, it is a set of guidelines for a hospital interested in implementing a compliance program to consider. The recommendations and guidelines provided in this document must be considered depending upon their applicability to each particular hospital.

This manual will assist organizations attempting to adopt the very principles and standards outlined by the OIG. This is accomplished by turning the structural concepts into written templates that capture the essence of what is called for in the *Guidance.*

Best-practice tip

A key tool provided in this manual can be found in the Appendix I (*OIG Compliance Guidance for Hospitals*). The entire document is included, on CD-ROM with a cross reference to templates provided in this manual. It is recommended that readers scan this Appendix early on to see how it can assist them in developing and enhancing their compliance program.

This book also delves deeply into the seven compliance elements, providing insight into related issues as well as policy templates to use as starting points in developing or revising compliance policies and procedures. The following should be noted about the templates:

- They provide starting points from which an organization can tailor them to its own culture, environment, and needs

- Not all policy templates may be appropriate for all organizations

- Each organization should consider the obligations that will be imposed on it once a policy is adopted, for it is better not to have a policy than to have one that is ignored or routinely violated

The employment of the various templates to develop policies and procedures does not create an effective compliance program. Effective compliance programs are dynamic and interactive. To be successful, a compliance program should establish a *culture* within an organization that promotes prevention, detection, and resolution of instances of misconduct including the violation of laws, regulations, and the organization's policies and procedures.

This requires an organization's employees be convinced of the seriousness of the compliance initiative. Compliance programs require support and participation by all employees in the organization—especially individuals in management positions and those on the governing body. Therefore, this manual should be used as a guide in the development and modification of a compliance program tailored to the unique needs and environment of the organization.

Scope of the compliance program and other compliance guidance

One of the most important decisions an organization faces is defining the scope of the compliance program.

Healthcare is clearly one of the most regulated sectors of the economy. The OIG *Compliance Program Guidance* is focused upon compliance with laws, regulations, and policies enforced and regulated by the Department of Health and Human Services (HHS). However, healthcare organizations are subject to numerous other regulatory and enforcement agencies, and they face other significant regulatory risks. Therefore, we recommend that governing boards and management adopt an enterprise-wide approach to compliance to ensure all regulatory risks are included.

This approach does not mean that the compliance officer takes responsibility for the resolution of all identified "compliance issues." It does, however, mean that the governing body and executive management have made a decision to establish a system of controls to identify and reduce the organization's most significant risks. We believe that this is a good business decision and that to do less leaves the board and management very vulnerable.

The following is a partial list of the federal regulatory agencies, enforcement agencies, and laws, in addition to the OIG and HHS, that are driving the healthcare compliance agenda and that should be considered in developing and operating the compliance program:

United States Sentencing Commission

The most potent force for the development of compliance programs came as the result of the creation of the United States Sentencing Commission in the 1980s. This commission developed *Compliance Guidelines for Organizations* (Guidelines) that are mandated in the sentencing process. These Guidelines have been followed by the OIG in their compliance guidance documents. The Guidelines apply to all organizations in all business sectors and represent a very serious set of standards for organizations that come under investigation by the federal government. In developing a compliance program, it is important to understand these underpinnings.

Since the Sentencing Commission Guidelines went into effect in June 1992, control of healthcare fraud and abuse has become an increasingly high priority for the federal government. In the early 1990s, the federal government made healthcare fraud and abuse a major enforcement priority.

More than 500 healthcare entities have signed Corporate Integrity Agreements (CIA) that include mandates for compliance programs. The healthcare industry has moved to invest in its own insurance policy to guard against the ravages of federal regulators who believe that they have identified abusive and fraudulent practices. The best policy available to this industry is compliance with the Sentencing Guidelines.

Compliance with the Guidelines not only helps prevent violations of the law but also protects those in violation of the law from serious—and sometimes fatal—financing consequences. The Guidelines were designed to create powerful new incentives for organizations to implement effective compliance programs to prevent, detect, and correct violations of the law.

By taking a "carrot and sledgehammer" approach to sentencing, the Guidelines provide powerful incentives for companies to establish compliance programs. They virtually mandate that the corporation and prosecutors become partners by making violations very costly for those who do not implement compliance programs.

The Guidelines promise no immunity from prosecution, but it is reasonable to expect that the existence of a bona fide compliance program would exert some favorable influence on prosecutorial discretion. Further, the compliance program must meet the requirements of the Guidelines to be considered for a reduction in culpability.

Although the Guidelines are very general, they require at a minimum that the organization exercise due diligence in establishing and implementing a compliance program. The bottom line is that the organization's actions must demonstrate that the organization is not indifferent to the law and has adopted a proactive plan for compliance.

Outside influences on compliance policies and procedures
The Joint Commission and compliance
The Joint Commission on Accreditation of Healthcare Organizations (formerly known as JCAHO, now The Joint Commission) although not a regulatory agency, does have a significant impact on the compliance arena.

The Joint Commission evaluates and accredits nearly 17,000 healthcare organizations and programs in the United States. It is an independent, not-for-profit organization that is the major standards-setting and accrediting body in healthcare. Since 1951, The Joint Commission has developed professionally based standards and evaluated the compliance of healthcare organizations against set benchmarks. Some of the more significant areas where Joint Commission activity overlaps with OIG and other compliance guidance involve calling for codes or standards of conduct.

FDA

The Federal Drug Administration (FDA) regulates one out of seven dollars spent in the United States. Its major impact is in medical pharmaceuticals and devices.

OSHA and ERISA

Many other regulatory agencies, such as the Occupational Safety and Health Administration (OSHA), and federal regulations, such as the Employee Retirement Income Security Act (ERISA), have an impact on healthcare organizations. In addition, an entire body of employment law relates to employees, covering such issues as protection against discrimination, unlawful harassment, wrongful discharge, and negligent hiring. An integrated compliance program should ensure coordination of all these risk-management and compliance activities.

HIPAA

The passage of the Health Insurance Portability and Accountability Act of 1996 (HIPAA) created a whole new body of mandatory compliance issues relating to privacy and security of protected patient-health information.

Sarbanes-Oxley Act

More recently, the Sarbanes-Oxley Act set new governance and compliance standards for publicly traded companies, and these standards are increasingly being applied to non-profit and non-publicly-traded healthcare entities.

Building consensus for the compliance program

Achieving consensus among the members of the management team and oversight board can be the most difficult step in moving forward with a compliance program. To take this step, both parties must understand that a commitment to building an effective compliance program is not based upon a negative decision or upon a decision to create a program simply because the government wants it done. Stressing the benefits of a compliance program can help promote this understanding.

The benefits of an effective compliance program include:

- Can dramatically reduce penalties if violations occur

- Improves internal communication and feedback to management

- Provides useful intelligence on the actual operations environment

- Reduces the likelihood of civil and criminal wrongdoing

- Ensures that legal/policy changes are disseminated quickly to all employees

- Reduces vulnerability and liability exposure to "whistle blowing"

- Improves crisis-response capabilities

- Alerts senior management—and permits quick and response—to emerging issues

- Reassures board/community that improper conduct is being addressed

- Promotes good business by having everyone adhere to the same rules

- Avoids having a compliance program imposed by enforcement agencies

Once the commitment is made by the governance board and management, the individual or committee responsible for the development and implementation is faced with a number of questions and decisions. To simplify the process, keep the following principles in mind:

- Effective compliance programs are tailored to the unique environment and needs of an individual organization and are not easily achieved through a cookie-cutter approach.

- Compliance programs should have behavioral objectives—changing or improving the culture of the organization so that employees will raise problems and concerns without fear of retaliation, and will trust management to address their issues appropriately.

- Compliance programs should build upon and coordinate existing compliance activities, such as existing auditing and monitoring actions, grievance procedures, and in-service training.

- Compliance programs should be broad in scope, sometimes referred to as "enterprise-wide," and should include all regulatory risks rather than being narrowly focused on a particular risk area, such as Medicare/Medicaid reimbursement.

Providing structure for corporate compliance programs

The OIG believes that every effective compliance program must begin with a formal commitment by all of the organization's governing body to include all of the applicable elements identified by them. They note that, at a minimum, comprehensive compliance programs should include the following seven elements:

1. Development and distribution of written standards of conduct, as well as written policies and procedures that promote the organization's commitment to compliance (e.g., by including adherence to compliance as an element in evaluating managers and employees). These documents should address specific areas of potential fraud, such as claims development and submission processes, code gaming, and financial relationships with physicians and other healthcare professionals.

2. Designation of a chief compliance officer and other appropriate bodies (e.g., a corporate compliance committee) who are charged with the responsibility of operating and monitoring the compliance program and who report directly to the CEO and the governing body.

3. Development and implementation of regular, effective education and training programs for all affected employees.

4. Maintenance of a process such as a hotline to receive complaints, and the adoption of procedures to protect the anonymity of complainants and to protect whistleblowers from retaliation.

5. Development of a system to respond to allegations of improper/illegal activities and the enforcement of appropriate disciplinary action against employees who have violated internal compliance policies, applicable statutes, regulations, or federal healthcare program requirements.

6. Use of audits and/or other evaluation techniques to monitor compliance and assist in the reduction of identified problem areas.

7. Investigation and remediation of identified systemic problems and the development of policies addressing the non-employment or retention of sanctioned individuals.

A framework for development of compliance program policies and procedures

As a healthcare organization begins to develop a corporate compliance program, it is essential to establish a framework for the individual(s) responsible for the program's operation and oversight. Once the compliance program begins functioning, policy statements should be issued to the organization related to areas of compliance risk. Compliance policy/procedures should address:

- Government expectations

- Establishing a framework for the compliance program

- Establishing an infrastructure for the compliance program

- Providing guidance on critical compliance-related areas

- Explaining compliance-office duties and responsibilities

- Providing specific guidance on areas of specific compliance risk

- Setting expectations for everyone in the work environment

- Assisting in avoiding violations of laws and regulations

Endnotes

1. See for example the OIG Compliance Program for Hospitals, 63 FR 8987 (Feb 23, 1998), OIG Supplemental Compliance Program Guidance for Hospitals, 70 FR 4958 (Jan. 31, 2005).

2. 2006 Federal Sentencing Guidelines Manual, Chapter 8, § 8B2.1 "Effective Compliance and Ethics Program". *www.ussc.gov/2006guid/8b2_1.html*. The USSC Web site posts the *Federal Sentencing Guidelines Manual*, as well as information about the USSC, other USSC publications, and federal sentencing statistics (*www.ussc.gov*).

3. Health Insurance Portability and Accountability Act of 1996 (HIPAA), Pub. L. 104-191.

4. The Sarbanes-Oxley Act of 2002 (Pub. L. No. 107-204, 116 Stat. 745), also known as the Public Company Accounting Reform and Investor Protection Act of 2002, is a United States federal statute signed into law on July 30, 2002 in response to a number of major corporate and accounting scandals including those affecting Enron, Tyco International, Peregrine Systems and WorldCom. See *49 Steps to Implement Sarbanes-Oxley Best Practices*, (AIS, 2006) for details on its application to the healthcare and non-profit sectors.

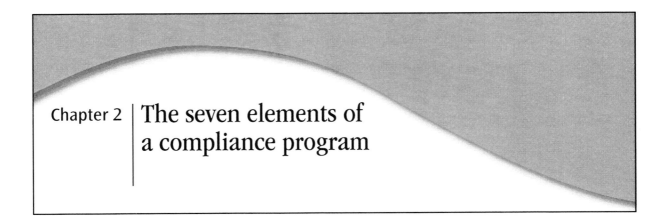

Chapter 2 | The seven elements of
a compliance program

Federal Sentencing Commission Guidelines for organizations[1]

In 1991, the United States Sentencing Commission promulgated guidelines to govern the imposition of
sentences by federal judges on organizational defendants. Referred to as the Federal Sentencing Guidelines for Organizations (FSGO, or Guidelines), the Guidelines impose harsh penalties upon organizations whose employees or other agents have committed federal crimes.

Penalties include:

- Restitution

- Remedial orders

- Community service

- Substantial fines, based upon a point system for determining severity of offense

The Guidelines encourage organizations to develop "effective programs to prevent and detect violations
of law" and prescribe seven "types of steps" that should be included in an effective program. Where
organizations demonstrate an effort to implement the seven steps, lower sanctions are levied by federal
judges.

The seven steps include the following:

1. Organizational implementation of compliance standards and procedures that are reasonably
   capable of reducing the prospect of criminal conduct

2. The assignment of high-level personnel to oversee compliance with such standards and procedures

3. Due care in avoiding delegation to individuals whom the organization knew, or should have known, had a propensity to engage in illegal activities

4. Communication of standards and procedures, by requiring participation in training programs or by disseminating publications that explain in a practical manner what is required

5. Establishing monitoring, auditing, and reporting systems by creating and publicizing a reporting system whereby employees and other agents can report criminal conduct without fear of retribution

6. Enforcing standards through appropriate mechanisms, including, as appropriate, discipline of individuals responsible for the failure to detect an offense

7. Developing appropriate responses to offenses by taking all reasonable steps to respond appropriately and to prevent further similar offenses, including any necessary modification of programs

These Guidelines apply to almost all types of organizations including corporations, partnerships, unions, not-for-profit organizations, and trusts. This includes healthcare entities such as hospitals, skilled nursing facilities, hospices, durable medical equipment suppliers, pharmaceutical manufacturers, pharmacies, physician practices, etc.

One significant aspect of the Guidelines is that each organization is responsible for the wrongful acts of its employees as long as the employees were acting in their official capacity. The theory is that each organization shares a degree of culpability if an employee acts in an unlawful manner, even if the organization did not know of, or approve of, their actions.

HHS Office of Inspector General's Compliance Guidance

Beginning in February 1997[2], the U.S. Department of Health and Human Services (HHS) Office of Inspector General (OIG) began adapting these seven steps or elements into its compliance guidance for hospitals.[3]

Subsequently, it issued similar guidance to other healthcare sectors.[4] The elements represent a guide—a process that can be used by hospitals large or small, urban or rural, for-profit or not-for-profit. Moreover, the elements can be incorporated into the managerial structure of multi-hospital, and integrated delivery, systems. These suggested guidelines can be tailored to fit the needs and financial realities of a particular hospital.

The OIG is cognizant that, with regard to compliance programs, one model is not suitable to every hospital. Nonetheless, the OIG believes every hospital, regardless of size or structure, can benefit from the principles espoused in this Guidance.

The OIG believes that every effective compliance program must begin with a formal commitment by the hospital's governing body to include all of the applicable recommended elements that expand on the seven steps of the Federal Sentencing Guidelines. At a minimum, the OIG states that a comprehensive compliance program should include the following seven elements:

1. The development and distribution of written standards of conduct, as well as written policies and procedures that promote the hospital's commitment to compliance (e.g., by including adherence to compliance as an element in evaluating managers and employees) and that address specific areas of potential fraud, such as claims development and submission processes, code gaming, and financial relationships with physicians and other healthcare professionals

2. The designation of a chief compliance officer and other appropriate bodies (e.g., a corporate compliance committee) charged with the responsibility of operating and monitoring the compliance program, and who report directly to the chief executive officer (CEO) and the governing body

3. The development and implementation of regular, effective education and training programs for all affected employees

4. The maintenance of a process such as a hotline to receive complaints, and the adoption of procedures to protect the anonymity of complainants and to protect whistleblowers from retaliation

5. The development of a system to respond to allegations of improper/illegal activities and the enforcement of appropriate disciplinary action against employees who have violated internal compliance policies, applicable statutes, regulations, or federal healthcare program requirements

6. The use of audits and/or other evaluation techniques to monitor compliance and assist in the reduction of identified problem areas

7. The investigation and remediation of identified systemic problems and the development of policies addressing the non-employment or retention of sanctioned individuals

OIG Supplemental Guidance for Hospitals[5]

On January 27, 2005, the OIG issued its final Supplemental Compliance Program Guidance for Hospitals (Supplemental Guidance) that supplements its initial 1998 Compliance Program Guidance for Hospitals (Compliance Guidance).

The focus of this new document was on fraud and abuse risk areas and on providing assistance in assessing the effectiveness of compliance programs. It further provides insight into current OIG perspective on these issue areas.

The OIG also sets forth auditing and monitoring standards, emphasizes the importance of evaluating the effectiveness of compliance programs through performing regular reviews, and identifies certain factors that effective compliance programs often contain.

The OIG expects hospitals and other entities in the health sector to review their compliance programs to ensure they accommodate the principles outlined by the Supplemental Guidance. Further, hospitals should ensure their auditing and monitoring processes address the risk areas specified in the Supplemental Guidance. Also, hospitals should conduct a compliance review of any relationships that potentially fall within the specified risk areas. (**Note:** These topics are covered in this manual in Chapter 2, Compliance Element 6, including templates 27–31.)

The factors that should be addressed in determining effectiveness of the compliance program include:

1. Designation of a compliance officer and committee (see Compliance Element 2, templates 3–15)

2. Development of compliance policies and procedures (see Written Policies and Procedures, template 1, as well as numerous other policy templates throughout this book and on the CD-ROM)

3. Open lines of communication within the hospital's organization (see Compliance Element 4, templates 17–20 among others)

4. Appropriate training and educating of hospital staff (see Compliance Element 3, template 16)

5. Conducting internal monitoring and auditing (see Compliance Element 6, Auditing and Monitoring, templates 27–31)

6. Consistently responding to detected deficiencies (see Compliance Elements 5 and 7, templates 21, 32, 33)

7. Enforcement of disciplinary standards (See Compliance Elements 5 and 7, templates 22–24)

The OIG's original Compliance Guidance was designed to assist hospitals in the development of an effective compliance program and to assist in developing systems to comply with the rules and regulations for participating in federal healthcare programs.

As with the initial Compliance Guidance, the OIG recognizes that compliance program implementation has become more sophisticated, requiring means to ensure that the program is functioning effectively. It emphasizes the importance of development and implementation of compliance policies and procedures, as well as tools for analyzing compliance with applicable laws and regulations. The OIG restates the recognition that there is no one way to develop and operate an effective compliance program.

The Supplemental Guidance suggests that each hospital implement a code of conduct (see template 2).

The Supplemental Guidance concludes by reminding hospitals of their obligation to the requirements for, and the benefits of, reporting a violation of compliance standards to the appropriate federal and state authorities within 60 days after determining that credible evidence of a violation exists (see Compliance Element 5, templates 25, 26).

By and large, the Supplemental Guidance does not expand on the identification of risk areas but rather includes substantial revisions to the section pertaining to arrangements between hospitals and those (particularly physicians) who are in a position to influence the flow of business (see Auditing and Monitoring). Two major enforcement-related statutes are cited, including the physician referral statute (the Stark Law) and the federal Anti-Kickback Statute (Anti-kickback). The Stark Law section provides a three-part inquiry for hospitals to use:

1. Is there a referral from a physician for designated health services (DHS)?

2. If so, does the physician (or an immediate family member) have a financial relationship with the entity furnishing the DHS?

3. If so, does the financial relationship fit an exception?

The OIG also addresses the definition of "financial relationship" and the necessity that hospitals meet all conditions of an exception to immunize them from violations of the Stark Law.

The federal Anti-Kickback Statute is assigned to the OIG exclusively for enforcement, both in terms of the criminal provisions and the administrative enforcement procedures.

In particular, the OIG identified these areas of risk under Anti-kickback:

- Joint ventures

- Compensation arrangements with physicians

- Relationships with other healthcare entities

- Recruitment arrangements

- Discounts

- Medical staff credentialing

- Malpractice insurance subsidies

The Supplemental Guidance includes a discussion of a hospital's responsibilities under the Emergency Medical Treatment and Active Labor Act (EMTALA). This discussion suggests that hospital policies clearly set forth when an individual must receive a medical screening examination to determine whether the individual is suffering from an emergency medical condition.

Also, the OIG discusses the procedure for transferring a patient with an emergency medical condition. Furthermore, the OIG suggests that hospitals educate their emergency department personnel and on-call physicians regarding their responsibilities under EMTALA.

Another key area of interest expressed by the OIG in the new Guidance is a reminder that the OIG has the ability to exclude a facility from participation in federal healthcare programs if the facility provides unnecessary or substandard care. They further warn hospitals of the dangers of providing remuneration to Medicare or Medicaid beneficiaries to attract their business. Such inducements include gifts and gratuities, cost-sharing waivers, and free transportation. Further, the OIG includes a brief discussion of a hospital's compliance with the privacy and security rules of the Health Insurance Portability and Accountability Act of 1996 (HIPAA).

Another warning offered in the Guidance is that hospitals should not routinely bill Medicare or Medicaid substantially more than they usually charge other payers. It is advisable to review this document in detail for other OIG insights on high-risk areas on compliance.

In all its compliance guidances, the OIG stresses the importance of an effective compliance program. The OIG makes it clear that adding compliance elements and steps without the compliance program being effective is no program at all.

In fact, such a "paint-by-the-numbers" approach might be considered a "sham" program. As a further note, the original Compliance Guidance for Hospitals used the term "effective" in various forms 19 times. Whenever a government document repeats something that many times, you can bet it means they are serious about it.

In the following pages, these seven elements presented in various forms by the Federal Sentencing Commission and OIG will be described in more detail and supplemented with templates that can assist in compliance program implementation and enhancement.

References

1. See 2006 Federal Sentencing Guidelines Manual, Chapter 8, § 8B2.1 "Effective Compliance and Ethics Program." *www.ussc.gov/2006guid/8b2_1.html*. The USSC Web site posts the Federal Sentencing Guidelines Manual, as well as information about the USSC, other USSC publications, and Federal sentencing statistics (*www.ussc.gov/2006guid/8b2_1.html.www.ussc.gov*).

2. Compliance Program Guidance for Clinical Laboratories PDF (63 FR 45076; August 24, 1998).*www.oig.hhs. gov/fraud/complianceguidancee.html*.

3. See for example the OIG Compliance Program for Hospitals (63 FR 8987; Feb 23, 1998), OIG Supplemental Compliance Program Guidance for Hospitals (70 FR 4958; Jan. 31, 2005).

4. Compliance Program Guidance for Home Health Agencies (63 FR 42410; August 7, 1998); Compliance Program Guidance for Third-Party Medical Billing Companies (63 FR 70138; December 18, 1998); Compliance Program Guidance for the Durable Medical Equipment Prosthetics, Orthotics, and Supply Industry (64 FR 36368; July 6, 1999); Compliance Program Guidance for Hospices (64 FR 54031; October 5, 1999); Final Compliance Program Guidance for Medicare+Choice Organizations (64 FR 61893;November 15, 1999); Final Compliance Program Guidance for Nursing Facilities (65 FR 14289; March 16, 2000); *Federal Register* Notice: Solicitation of Information and Recommendations for Developing a Compliance Risk Guidance for the Ambulance Industry; Final Compliance Program Guidance for Individual and Small Group Physician Practices (65 *FR* 59434; October 5, 2000); Final Compliance Program Guidance for Ambulance Supplers; Complaince Program Guidance for Pharmaceutical Manufacturers 04/28/03. All available at the HHS OIG Web site, *www.oig.hhs.gov/ fraud/complianceguidance*.

5. Office of Inspector General Supplemental Compliance Program Guidance for Hospitals (70 *FR* 4958; Jan. 31, 2005). Can also be found at the HHS OIG Web site: *www.oig.hhs.gov/fraud/complianceguidance.html*.

Compliance Element 1: Written standards, code of conduct, and written policies and procedures

Fundamental to any successful compliance program is providing written guidance for all affected parties as to what is expected of them in the work place. A significant part of this book will be devoted to providing templates and materials that can be used in developing this guidance.

Generally speaking, guidance begins at the top, with the mission and vision statements of the organization. These are the basic guiding principles for employees and those who deal with the entity.

After that are general expectations and guidelines as to how individuals in the workplace are expected to behave consistent with these principles. These are known as the standards, or code, of conduct. It is the keystone or "constitution" of an effective compliance program. Specific written guidance comes in the form of published policies and procedures that guide individuals performing various activities.

The mission/vision statements, code, and policy documents should all be consistent. It will not serve an organization well to have standards of conduct that are inconsistent with the written policies and procedures of the organization. Consequently, new code and policy development should be referenced to ensure internal consistency.

Most organizations and entities have developed their own mission/vision statements specific to their culture and business sectors. As such, this book will not address that subject, other than to note that many organizations revisit those principles in light of corporate compliance program development. It may stimulate revisions or enhancements in those statements.

The first element of a compliance program addresses guidance in the form of codes, or standards, of conduct, and compliance policies. The office of Inspector General (OIG) refers to policies throughout all seven elements of an effective compliance program. As such, a major portion of the book will involve the discussion of, and templates for, policy documents. This book strongly encourages that all aspects of the compliance program be founded in written policy guidance. This will serve many purposes, including:

- Ensuring internal consistency in the compliance program and expected behavior (business, professional, and personal conduct)

- Providing tangible evidence of the development of the compliance program in the organization

- Facilitating oversight by the compliance officer, senior management, and the board of directors on the progress of compliance program development

- Establishing benchmarks (internal controls) by which ongoing auditing and monitoring for compliance can be made

Before diving into compliance program development, it is important to address what these policy documents should look like in general. Therefore, this subject will be touched upon before addressing the question of codes, or standards, of conduct (collectively, the code). This approach will allow the writer to decide whether issues related to the code should be included in written policy guidance.

Written policies and procedures

The OIG at the U.S. Department of Health and Human Services (HHS) has issued a number of compliance program guidance documents. They are an elaboration on the Federal Sentencing Commission "Guidelines for Organizations" as applied to the healthcare industry.

The OIG notes that every compliance program should require the development and distribution of written compliance policies that identify specific areas of risk to the organization. They call for the policies to be developed and reviewed annually under the direction and supervision of operations management.

Those policies related to the organization and operation of the corporate compliance program are to be developed and reviewed annually under the direction and supervision of the corporate compliance officer. Furthermore, compliance-related policies should be provided to all individuals who are affected by the particular policy at issue. The OIG also suggests that the compliance officer and the corporate compliance committee have an opportunity to review and comment on such policies prior to final approval.

Compliance policies fall into two general categories:

1. Those that relate to the operation of the compliance program.

2. Those that relate to specific areas of compliance risk.

3. In the former, the compliance officer bears the responsibility for the development, implementation, management, and enforcement of the policies. In the latter, the development, implementation, management, and enforcement of the policies fall on the operations' managers responsible for the risk area, with oversight by the compliance officer.

In both cases, the policies should be developed under the direction and supervision of the compliance officer and the compliance committee. Once developed, the policies should be disseminated to all individuals affected by the particular policy at issue, and appropriate training and monitoring should be conducted.

Providing a framework for policy development

Compliance policy development can be a very difficult and sometimes contentious process. Depending on where people are in an organization, they will have differing views on what should be reduced to written guidance and how that guidance should be presented to the work force. It is therefore advisable to develop and establish an agreed-upon specific set of protocols that ensure uniformity, consistency, and management support in policy development. Proper dissemination of all approved policies can then be made.

Before moving to develop compliance policies for any particular subject, it is advisable to establish a process, form, and format for policy development. Establishing the formalities of how proposed policy documents will be presented, and the process that will be followed in gaining approval, will likely prevent a lot of problems later. When proposed policies are finally presented, the issues of focus will be substantive, not procedural.

Best-practice tip

Develop a process, format, and form for compliance policy documents before beginning work on a specific policy issue. This will ensure that future compliance policy development will remain focused on the substantive issues rather that on procedural ones.

In order to take this step, it is important to decide on the form and format of the compliance policy documents. They should be consistent in organization, and recognizable. It is recommended that the policy document consist of seven elements:

1. Header Block

2. Background Introduction

3. Purpose/Objectives Statement

4. Definitions Section

5. Policy Statements

6. Procedures

7. References

Header block

The title should clearly identify the general topic of the policy and assist those who may be searching for guidance on the policy's topic area. The header block should also include, but not necessarily be limited to:

- The title of the policy

- Identity of the department responsible for drafting, reviewing, and enforcing the policy

- Effective date of the policy

- Policy number

- Date of approval

- Identity of approval authority

- Whether it replaces or modifies an existing policy

- Number of pages included in the document

Background section

This can be used to introduce the context for the policy document. If the policy relates to a specific law, regulation, or compliance standard, this section can explain how the policy document is designed to address that issue.

In short, it can put the policy in context. It can also be used to relate and/or differentiate the particular policy document to other written guidance. This section should assist in understanding and following the policy. It is best to have this precede the statement of purpose.

Purpose/Objective section

When developing or revising a policy, begin with a statement-of-purpose section that defines the intent and objectives of the policy. It should be relatively short and direct. It is suggested that it begin with an active verb, such as, "to promote . . . , to comply . . . , to ensure . . . ," etc.

Definitions

In many cases, terminology will be used that requires understanding and clarification in order to meet the intention of the policy document. In those cases, a special section of the policy document should be used to provide definition in the context that is used in the document. These may be of a legal nature or may be specific to the organization. It is advisable to cite the authority for the definitions being used.

Policy statement

This section should include general statements describing the goals to be met by the implementation of the policy.

Procedures statement

This section should clearly define the specific tasks required to address the purpose and objectives of the policy in a step-by-step format.

References

This section can be used for legal and regulatory citations, as well as that of the organization. If the policy document was created in response to legal or regulatory authority, that authority should be noted, along with a list of supporting and source documentation used to validate the policy and procedure. This also can be used to refer to other policy-related documents.

In drafting policy documents, sentences should be declarative, in the active voice, succinct, focused, and simple. Those policy documents related to the management and operation of the compliance program should be drafted by the compliance office before being sent forward for review and adoption. The department manager and other appropriate operations management personnel should review and comment on those draft policies and procedures addressing an identified compliance risk affecting their areas of responsibilities prior to review and approval by the executive compliance committee.

The compliance officer, in consultation with the compliance committee—and, as required, legal counsel—should coordinate development of all draft compliance program policies, and be responsible for submitting them to appropriate management and executives for review and comment prior to approval by the compliance committee, the chief executive officer (CEO), and, when appropriate, the board of directors.

In submitting the draft policies for approval, the compliance officer should include with the proposed policy and procedure a presentation of the compliance issues in question, a description of how the policy and procedure proposes to address such issues, and a plan for implementation (including any training required).

It is recommended that the compliance officer distribute the proposed policy and procedure, with justification, to the CEO and compliance committee members prior to the scheduled compliance committee meeting where approval will be sought.

The primary author/proponent of the policy and procedure should be prepared to make a presentation to the CEO and compliance committee describing the compliance issues in question, a description of how the policy and procedure will address them, and the plan for implementation. The CEO and compliance committee will hear the presentation of the policy and procedure for approval, implementation, and distribution.

Best-practice tip

The same process for submitting new policies and procedures should be followed for presenting a revision or modification to an existing policy document. To eliminate an existing operational compliance policy, it is advisable for the responsible department manager to make a written request to the compliance officer that includes the reason for the proposed action, and thereafter the proposal will be submitted to the compliance committee following the same procedure as described for new policies and procedures.

If the policy is one assigned to the compliance officer, then the compliance officer will present the justification directly to the compliance committee. All rescinded policies should be moved to a section designated for retired policies and procedures and filed by date. They should **NOT** be deleted from the records system or manuals.

In order to meet the suggested standards offered by the OIG, there should be an annual policy review by each department. This review should identify all compliance risks and whether a new policy or amended policy is needed to address that risk area. The review should also address the adequacy of all current compliance-related policies and procedures relevant to their area of responsibility.

The results of the reviews should be directed to the compliance officer, along with any proposed revisions, and new policies. Likewise, the compliance officer will review all compliance program policies annually and make appropriate recommendations for revisions or new policies in accordance with this policy. The compliance officer, working with departmental managers, should ensure proper dissemination, education, and training of approved new and revised policies to all affected parties.

On the accompanying CD-ROM, we've included a sample Template 1: Policy development and implementation policy (Template 2-1-1) designed to transform the advice above into a policy template. It is advisable to consider development and implementation of a "policy-development policy" as the first step in compliance policy development, with all other policies developed according to the protocols established by this policy.

Code of conduct

The term "standards of conduct" refers to written guidance for employees on expected behavior in the workplace. Organizations use a variety of titles for their standards of conduct, including "code of conduct," "code of business ethics," and "code of ethics," among others. In fact, the OIG frequently interchanges "standards of conduct" and "code of conduct." Code of conduct is used in this book as the generic term for all these variations. By whatever title, it should:

- Articulate the organization's commitment to comply with all criminal, civil, and administrative laws, with an emphasis on preventing fraud and abuse

- Describe conduct that could give rise to a liability for the organization, particularly a legal or regulatory liability to the federal government

- Provide employees with a clear understanding of what is expected in the workplace, and form the basis for compliance training and education

At the earliest opportunity, whoever has been given the responsibility for code of conduct development should initiate a plan to organize a compliance workgroup to assist in the process. He and she should also take responsibility for widely circulating the draft code of conduct document for comments and approval. This will be very important. Issuing a code of conduct without gaining internal support from all stakeholders—including employees, management, governing body, and physicians (if the organization provides medical services)—is risky.

The work group should operate under the direction of the compliance officer or designated corporate individual responsible for building the compliance program. It will be his or her responsibility to hammer it out, put the organization's mark on the code of conduct, and provide evidence of his or her involvement in creating the code.

Members of the workgroup should include representatives from legal counsel, human resources, finance/audit, and the various operational areas. If the organization delivers healthcare services, then medical/clinical representation should be included on the group as well.

The OIG Compliance Program Guidance documents contain 13 specific references that offer insight on what is expected in a code. The OIG-suggested elements for a code of conduct include the following:

- Articulate the commitment to comply with all federal and state standards

- Emphasize preventing fraud and abuse

- State mission, goals, and ethical requirements of compliance

- Clearly express that it applies to governing body members, officers, managers, employees, physicians, affiliated providers operating under the organization's control, and, where appropriate, contractors and other agents

- Include a statement of management's commitment to compliance

- Cover the non-retaliation policy, problem-resolution process, and the hotline

- Include a clear commitment to quality of care, and recognize that a potential benefit of a compliance program is to improve the quality of patient care

- Specifically address billing, coding, the Anti-Kickback Statute, and other legal Medicare and Medicaid fraud and abuse issues

---

Best-practice tip

The code should also address human resource issues, such as sexual harassment, wrongful discharge, abusive labor practices, discrimination, etc., in that failure to comply with human resource–related laws, regulations, and policies can easily give rise to serious liabilities.

OIG compliance guidance provides suggestions on code development and distribution, including the following:

- The code development process is critical because it must be acceptable by senior management and frontline employees.

- The code also must be consistent with the organization's underlying policies.

- It is important to show evidence of top-down commitment to the code development process. Therefore, the executive compliance committee established to advise the compliance officer and assist in the implementation of the compliance program (or a subgroup thereof) should participate in developing the code.

- The code should be approved by the organization's governing body.

- The code should be written in language that is readily understood by everyone in the workplace. Technical language and legalese should especially be avoided in sections dealing with complex legal and regulatory requirements.

- It should be distributed to all employees.

- It should be regularly updated as applicable statutes, regulations, and federal healthcare program requirements are modified.

Best-practice tip

Include a CEO letter in the code of conduct that:
- Affirms the support of senior management and the governing body for the code of conduct and the company compliance program
- Encourages reporting of wrongdoing
- Warrants no retribution/retaliation for reporting
- Allows anonymity and confidentiality to those who report

As the cornerstone of the compliance program, the code of conduct is the responsibility of the compliance officer and the organization's oversight bodies. Although developed inclusively, the compliance officer should guide the development and approval process, as well as ensure that it is periodically reviewed and updated as appropriate. For this reason, a policy outlining specific responsibilities for code development, approval, revision, and distribution is essential to an effective compliance program.

TEMPLATE 2:

CODE (STANDARDS) OF CONDUCT

DEPARTMENT: Compliance Office	EFFECTIVE DATE:
POLICY NUMBER:	APPROVAL DATE:
POLICY: Code (Standards) of Conduct Policy	APPROVED BY:
POLICY REPLACED:	NUMBER OF PAGES:

BACKGROUND

U.S. Department of Health and Human Services (HHS) Office of Inspector General (OIG) compliance guidance recommends that compliance programs include the development of a written code of conduct that includes a clearly delineated commitment to compliance by management, employees, affiliated providers, vendors, and contractors operating under control of the organization.

PURPOSE

We are committed to conducting business ethically and in conformance with all applicable laws and regulations. The purpose of this policy document is to provide guidance on the development and dissemination of the organization's code of conduct.

DEFINITION

The term "code of conduct" refers to the written guidance on standards of conduct and expected behavior of employees and others in the workplace.

POLICY

We will maintain and periodically update a written code of conduct to provide guidance on employee and organizational responsibilities related to compliance and to address specific issues related to quality of care, reimbursement, financial relationships, and other critical areas, with a particular emphasis on preventing fraud and abuse.

1. The code of conduct will address important parts of the compliance program including but not limited to employee and management responsibilities, the problem-resolution process, employee hotline, and non-retaliation policy. It will also address specific issues related to quality of care, reimbursement, financial relationships, and other critical areas.

2. All employees will receive a copy of the code of conduct and participate in periodic training sessions that include a thorough review of the code of conduct.

3. The compliance officer will have primary responsibility for developing and periodically updating the code of conduct.

PROCEDURES

1. The executive compliance committee and the audit and board of director's compliance committee will be responsible for oversight and final approval of the code of conduct.

2. The code will be written at a basic reading level, avoiding complex or legal language.

3. The code of conduct will address the following critical areas related to compliance:

   - Define those who are covered by the code of conduct

   - Organization's mission and values

   - Quality of care/service

   - Compliance with laws and regulations

   - Human resource practices

   - Billing, coding, claims processing, vouchering, etc.

   - Protection and use of information, property, and assets

   - Conflicts of interest

   - Health and safety

   - Duty to follow laws and report suspected, potential, or known violations

   - Reporting options/channels available to employees, including the hotline

   - Responsibilities of supervisors and managers

   - Non-retaliation policy

3. The code of conduct will be distributed to all board members, executives, managers, employees, and those with whom business is conducted, as appropriate. Copies will also be provided to all new employees as part of their orientation. Recipients will sign a statement acknowledging:

   - Receipt

   - Reading and understanding its contents

   - Agreeing to abide by its provisions

4. All employees receive training on the code of conduct to help them understand how it applies to everyday work situations. The compliance officer will ensure that documentation is maintained as evidence that those employees have received training.

5. The compliance officer will investigate possible violations of the code of conduct and ensure that appropriate disciplinary or corrective action is taken when necessary.

REFERENCES/CITATIONS

OIG Compliance Program Guidance for Hospitals published by the Office of Inspector General in a *Federal Register* notice, dated February 23, 1998, and Supplemental Compliance Guidance January 31, 2005 (see 70 *FR* 4858, available at OIG Web site: *http://oig.hhs.gov/authorities/docs/cpghosp.pdf.*)

Federal Sentencing Guidelines Manual, 2003 version can be found at *www.ussc.gov/2003guid/TABCON03.htm.*

"Corporate Responsibility and Corporate Compliance: A Resource for Health Care Boards of Directors," published by the OIG, in conjunction with the American Health Lawyers Association.

Compliance Element 2: Compliance officer/other appropriate bodies

Board leadership and oversight

An effective compliance program must be a "top-down" program, beginning with the board of directors (board) and followed by the chief executive officer (CEO), president, chief operating officer (COO), and so on, through the executive and management structure of the organization down to the lowest echelon of employees. Top-down leadership for compliance programs has been a consistent theme in government guidance documents. Both the Department of Justice and the Department of Health and Human Services (HHS) Office of Inspector General (OIG) recommend that the board be intimately involved in providing ongoing oversight of compliance efforts.

In addition, according to the OIG, a comprehensive compliance program should include the designation of appropriate bodies (e.g., a corporate compliance committee) charged with the responsibility of operating and monitoring the compliance program, and who report directly to the CEO and the governing body. Building a structure that recognizes this is a very important part of any credible compliance effort.

For years, OIG compliance guidance documents have emphasized that the compliance effort of any organization begins with the board. This is consistent with a long history of legal expectation for boards arising from fiduciary duties, derivative suits, good-faith standards, etc. The OIG compliance guidance documents are designed to assist governing bodies in the proper management and operation of an organization. They call upon corporate officers to provide ethical leadership to the organization and to ensure that adequate systems are in place to facilitate ethical and legal conduct.

The OIG recognizes in its guidance documents that adopting and implementing an effective compliance program requires a substantial commitment of time, energy, and resources by the governing body. In response to the OIG guidance, many organizations have expanded their traditional audit committee into an audit *and* compliance committee to include compliance oversight.

Corporate responsibility and corporate compliance

A guidance document published jointly by the OIG and the American Health Lawyers Association (AHLA) addresses the importance of board involvement. This guidance, entitled "Corporate Responsibility and Corporate Compliance: A Resource for Health Care Boards of Directors," reinforces the criticality of leadership and oversight.

The "Corporate Responsibility and Corporate Compliance" document's stated purpose is to aid healthcare organization directors in asking knowledgeable and appropriate questions related to healthcare corporate compliance. The document focuses on the "duty of care" and again cites the Caremark case. It also notes directors' duties with respect to both development and oversight of compliance programs.

The OIG identifies two distinct contexts for this: decision-making functions and oversight functions. It goes on to offer a list of suggested questions that board members should ask in each arena.

As the OIG has repeatedly stated, case law suggests that the failure of a corporate director to attempt, in good faith, to institute a compliance program in certain situations may be a breach of a director's fiduciary obligation. They cite the Caremark case as an example.[2]

The Caremark case alleged that directors breached their fiduciary duties by failing to effectively monitor the conduct of employees who violated various state and federal laws regarding payments to healthcare providers. This case ultimately led to the organization pleading guilty to criminal charges and paying substantial penalties.

The chancellor in the case concluded that a director does have a general duty to ensure that there is an effective compliance and control system in place. The case further showed that the failure to do so could, under some circumstances, "render a director liable for losses caused by non-compliance with applicable legal standards."

The duty of care argument further calls for reasonable inquiry of management to obtain information necessary to ensure compliance with applicable laws and regulations. It was recognized that the board is not expected to know everything about a topic they are asked to consider. Where justified, they may rely on the advice of management and of outside advisors, attorneys, and consultants.

The AHLA and OIG make it clear in the guidance document that there are two separate obligations with respect to the duty of care: one for a specific decision or a particular board action, and the other for providing oversight of the day-to-day business operations, including compliance with applicable laws and regulations. The board's obligations with respect to corporate compliance programs arise within the context of that oversight function.

In providing oversight, the board has a duty to attempt in good faith to ensure that:

- Adequate information and reporting systems exist

- The reporting system is adequate to assure the board that appropriate information regarding compliance with applicable laws will come to its attention in a timely manner as a matter of ordinary operations

As such, failure by a board to reasonably oversee the implementation of a compliance program may put the organization at risk and, under extraordinary circumstances, expose individual members to personal liability for losses caused by the corporate non-compliance.

The duty of care does not mean that it is a board's responsibility to conduct investigations or internal inquiries concerning compliance with laws and regulations. That responsibility lies with management and, more particularly, with the compliance officer. It does mean that there is a duty to ensure that potential violations that surface are being addressed by management. If, on the other hand, there is a major red flag of a material nature (financial improprieties or fraud), board members should satisfy themselves that the issues are being addressed promptly and competently.

In 2007, once again the OIG and the AHLA developed new and reinforcing guidance on this subject.[3] They noted that:

> The basic fiduciary duty of care principle, which requires a director to act in good faith with the care an ordinarily prudent person would exercise under similar circumstances, is being tested in the current corporate climate. Embedded within the duty of care is the concept of reasonable inquiry. In other words, directors are expected to make inquiries to management to obtain the information necessary to satisfy their duty of care.

This document also notes that boards of healthcare organizations increasingly are called to respond to oversight with respect to how quality of care affects matters of reimbursement and payment, efficiency, cost controls, and collaboration between organizational providers and individual and group practitioners. In the hospital setting, OIG and AHGLA note that the board duty includes:

- The conduct of the hospital as an institution

- Ensuring that the medical staff is accountable to the governing board for the quality of care provided to patients

- The maintenance of standards of professional care within the facility and requiring that the medical staff function competently

To underscore its view on board oversight, the OIG also encouraged Congress to increase its authority in dealing with boards and board members who are derelict in their oversight responsibilities. The passage of the Health Insurance Portability and Accountability Act of 1996 (HIPAA)[4] was a response to this plea. It states, in part:

> Any individual who has a direct or indirect ownership or control interest in a sanctioned entity and who knows or should know . . . of the action constituting the basis for the conviction or exclusion . . . ; or (ii) who is an officer or managing employee . . . of such an entity . . .

Thus, through HIPAA, the OIG has the authority to exclude board members from the healthcare industry if they knew or should have known about the activity that gave rise to a conviction or exclusion in the organization. This is the gross-negligent standard, and the OIG has the authority to administratively impose the sanction. It does not require judicial determination in the federal courts.

The significance of all of this recent activity is not only the willingness of the OIG to assist boards in carrying out their fiduciary obligations but also a warning that the OIG is willing to hold boards to these standards. This is not a hollow threat—the HIPAA authorities exist to give the OIG teeth to take action against board members who forget their fiduciary responsibilities. On July 30, 2002, the Sarbanes-Oxley Act of 2002 (SOX) (Public Law 107-204) was signed into law and is still being phased in among covered entities. It came as a result of some of the largest financial scandals in the nation's history. The SOX focused on a number of failures and corrective action measures mandated as a result. Among the major failures were several at the board level. As such, they received considerable attention. Although the SOX is limited to "covered entities" (that is, publicly traded companies), key principles from the legislation are moving to the healthcare sector.

In "Corporate Responsibility and Corporate Compliance: A Resource for Health Care Boards of Directors," the fiduciary role, duties, and obligations of board members are clarified through a number of suggested questions that organizations may ask related to both the structure of the compliance program and its operation. A checklist of questions for compliance officers and compliance committees to consider when developing a facility compliance program is located on the CD-ROM (Figure 2-2-1). This book will address these issues, both in terms of the board-level templates and in terms of other policy templates included in other sections of this book.

It makes best sense to begin compliance efforts at the top of the organization, at the board level and senior management. It is critical to gain buy-in from these levels. Without such buy-in, success in applying the principles of the SOX is likely to be very limited.

The board and CEO need to set the tone and provide the commitment to the effort. The smaller the organization, the more critical this step becomes in that the actions of the board and CEO are more visible to a larger percentage of management and the work force. the following steps to get the program underway.

An effective compliance program beginning at the top should include the creation at the board level of a compliance committee. The nomenclature can be decided by each organization. Establishing a committee at the executive level provides the necessary level of commitment to ensure proper development and implementation of a compliance effort that can be effective.

It must be an ongoing effort. It is a logical step in managing the implementation process. However, it is also important to everything else that follows. For this reason, it is placed as the first step in implementation, with each subsequent step following specific provisions of law.

The board of directors is the apex of any effective compliance program and is ultimately responsible for its proper implementation and continued operation. Privately held companies and nonprofit organizations whose directors are not truly independent should consider adding such independent directors to the board, to serve not only on the audit committee but also on a compensation committee that deals with management compensation (including bonuses and options to management shareholders).

It is assumed that an organization using this book has established (or is in the process of establishing) a compliance office and a compliance officer. The size and financial resources of an organization will necessarily dictate whether a full-time compliance officer can be appointed and a separate compliance office established.

> ### Best-practice tip
> Independent directors should constitute a simple majority or better of the board in order to exert strong and independent influence and oversight of both financial and program compliance.

If a full commitment is impossible or impractical due to limited size and financial resources, the organization should allocate resources and personnel on a part-time basis for compliance efforts. According to the OIG, "all healthcare organizations, regardless of size, location, or corporate structure, can establish an effective compliance program."[5]

Federal regulators and the public see the board as having major responsibilities in ensuring the existence of adequate internal controls of the corporation. This includes the accounting and financial systems, as well as proper auditing oversight of the corporation.

To be viewed as effective, board members must demonstrate they are objective, capable, and inquisitive, as well as evince a working knowledge of the entity's activities and environment. Board members are expected to commit the time necessary to fulfill their board responsibilities. The board is responsible for holding management accountable through its governance, guidance, and oversight activities. By selecting management, the board has, in effect, defined what it expects with regard to integrity and ethical values, and it must confirm its expectations through its oversight role. To do less, or to discharge these activities poorly, invites stockholder suits and investigations that may target board members.

Board oversight responsibilities

- Compliance with applicable laws, regulations, and policies

- Accurate and reliable accounting, auditing, and claims processing

- Compliance program development and implementation

- Adherence to high business standards, as well as legal and personal ethics

- Adequate compliance education, training, and communication

- Development, approval, and dissemination of a code of conduct

- Compliance policies/procedures developed and disseminated

Board-level audit and compliance committee

As early as 1940, the Securities and Exchange Commission encouraged the use of audit committees composed of independent directors to objectively assess the adequacy of financial reporting and internal controls. It was believed that management may face pressures to satisfy stakeholder expectations. Often these pressures related to compensation incentives, which might promote self-interest rather than the promotion of long-term organizational interest. An independent audit committee with adequate resources was seen as a means to overcome this problem.

This reliance on effective audit-committee oversight has grown over the years. Audit committees are now one of the focal points for remedying recent abuses in both the financial and the regulatory compliance arena. As a result, there has been a trend in expanding the role of these committees to include regulatory and legal compliance beyond financial reporting and internal controls. The OIG has expressed the opinion that every effective compliance program must begin with a formal commitment by the organization's governing body. The OIG guidance states,

> as a first step, a good faith and meaningful commitment on the part of the . . . administration, especially the governing body and the CEO, will substantially contribute to a program's successful implementation.

The OIG also sees effective board oversight of compliance as one of the board's critical fiduciary responsibilities. Many organizations have assigned compliance oversight responsibilities to the audit committee, changing the committee's name to the audit and compliance committee.

From the OIG viewpoint, the audit and/or compliance committee should provide oversight to the compliance program relating to the conduct of business that will ensure high ethical standards are met and that the mission, values, and code of conduct are properly communicated to all employees on an annual basis. In addition, it should provide oversight for the implementation of the compliance program and ensure adherence to the code of conduct and government rules/regulations.

Best-practice tip

Create an audit and compliance committee with responsibility for overseeing the compliance program, along with reviewing high-risk areas and internal controls.

The committee should also review the activities of management and its employees in light of the code of conduct and the compliance program to ensure that policies and procedures are properly understood and followed. Pursuant to guidance documents issued by the OIG, many healthcare organizations have adopted an audit and compliance committee that addresses financial as well as program compliance issues.

The board compliance committee, working with the compliance officer and entire management team, should take steps to ensure that ongoing auditing and monitoring of high-risk areas and compliance program administration are properly executed, documented, and in evidence.

The full board is responsible for selecting members for the audit and compliance committee. Such a committee generally includes three to five members. To be viewed as truly independent and effective, the majority of members should be independent or outside directors.

For the committee to be considered credible by oversight agencies and the public, its members should have diverse, complementary backgrounds with broad business knowledge, intelligence, and judgment. Familiarity with accounting principles, particularly for the committee chairman, is not only highly desirable but considered mandatory where accounting and financial issues play a large role in corporate governance and oversight.

Best-practice tip

All the members of the audit and compliance committee should be independent directors.

An audit and compliance committee of the board of directors, of the type described here, is fast becoming a critical element for any effective compliance program. The modern-day audit and compliance committee is expected to be diverse and able to do a lot of things. It must be able to hold the CEO accountable to benchmarks developed to support a strategy for having an effective compliance program.

Members of the audit committee must satisfy their required "duty of care." Stated broadly, that duty requires members of an audit and compliance committee to undertake a "reasonable inquiry" to ensure that they are fully informed of all relevant facts related to financial management, internal controls, adherence to regulatory standards, and development of the compliance program.

It is recommended the committee meet at least four times a year, with additional meetings held as necessary to discharge the committee's responsibilities. Written agendas for meetings should be prepared and minutes of meetings taken and provided to the board of directors to keep the board apprised of the committee's activities and recommendations. Sound procedures would result in the preparation of a formal annual report to the board of directors, summarizing the activities, conclusions, and recommendations during the past year, and the committee's agenda for the next year.

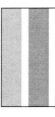

Best-practice tip

Establish/formalize procedures for regular meetings, with detailed minutes to document the committee's activities and recommendations.

In order for an audit and compliance committee to carry out all of its responsibilities, it should have financially literate members who are able to deal with the audit side of their oversight responsibilities. However, the committee should also understand the general standards and requirements concerning the development and implementation of an effective compliance program.

The development of an effective committee does not end with member appointments. However members of the committee should be willing to make the time commitments necessary to meet their obligations. They should undergo appropriate orientation relating to their duties, as well as briefings on industry and regulatory developments.

The audit and compliance committees should provide a forum separate from management in which the compliance officer and auditors can candidly review and discuss concerns. By doing this, the committee can help ensure that management properly supports the compliance program, development of sound system of internal controls, and implementation of policies and procedures promoting sound and lawful practices. This requires considerable interaction with the compliance officer, as well as with the financial officers and internal and external auditors.

Best-practice tip

Promote development of formal educational programs for board directors that include the business operations of the organization, review of internal control obligations, regulatory update, compliance and financial oversight responsibilities, etc.

Best-practice tip

The audit and compliance committee should meet periodically with the compliance officer and others responsible for regulatory and financial compliance during the course of the year in order to facilitate their oversight responsibilities.

The audit and compliance committee's role should be specifically addressed. It is clear that the role for this kind of board committee has been rapidly expanding. With the focus on "fiduciary responsibility" and "duty of care," the committee should be empowered with sufficient flexibility to perform its duties. The definition of the committee's role should also include a discussion of the committee structure, activities, and reporting requirements. This should be done through a formalized process that fully describes the duties and responsibilities of the committee.

Best-practice tip

Establish a board policy document that defines the duties and responsibilities for an audit and compliance committee.

The following template includes compliance oversight responsibilities only. If the organization prefers one comprehensive policy that incorporates both compliance and audit responsibilities, the template language could be incorporated into a broader policy statement.

References

1. "Corporate Responsibility and Corporate Compliance: A Resource for Health Care Boards of Directors," The Office of Inspector General of the U.S. Department of Health and Human Services, and the American Health Lawyers Association (2003). "An Integrated Approach to Corporate Compliance: A Resource for Health Care Organizations Boards of Directors," The Office of Inspector General of the U.S. Department of Health and Human Services; and the American Health Lawyers Association (2004).

2. In re Caremark International Inc. Derivative Litigation, 698 A. 2d 959 (Del. Ch. 1996).

3. "Corporate Responsibility and Health Care Quality: A Resource for Health Care Boards of Directors," The Office of Inspector General of the U.S. Department of Health and Human Services; and the American Health Lawyers Association, (2007).

4. (Public Law 104–191—Aug. 21, 1996, 110 STAT. 2005). Section 213 of that act, entitled, "Permissive Exclusion of Individuals with Ownership or Control Interest in Sanctioned Entities."

5. See The Office of Inspector General's Compliance Program Guidance for Hospitals.

TEMPLATE 3:

BOARD AUDIT AND COMPLIANCE COMMITTEE

DEPARTMENT: BOARD	EFFECTIVE DATE:
POLICY NUMBER:	APPROVAL DATE:
POLICY: Compliance Oversight by board Audit and Compliance Committee	APPROVED BY:
POLICY REPLACED:	NUMBER OF PAGES:

BACKGROUND

The Office of Inspector General (OIG) believes that board leadership and oversight are essential to the successful implementation of a corporate compliance program. In its compliance program guidance documents, the OIG promotes the designation of a board committee to provide proper oversight for the compliance program.

We are committed to the proper oversight of our corporate compliance program and have therefore assigned this responsibility to the audit and compliance committee of the board of directors.

PURPOSE

To provide guidance on the compliance oversight responsibilities of the audit and compliance committee of the board of directors.

POLICY

1. The board has established an audit and compliance committee charged with the responsibility of providing oversight for the audit and compliance of the organization and of ensuring the organization has adopted and implemented policies and procedures that will ensure compliance with all applicable laws, regulations, and policies.

2. The compliance committee will review and address matters relating to the compliance program. In so doing, it will:

- Assist the board of directors in fulfilling its responsibilities relating to legal and financial compliance with applicable laws, regulatory requirements, industry guidelines, and policies

- Provide a vehicle for communication between the board and management with respect to compliance

- Make recommendations to the full board that will assist the organization in conducting its activities in full compliance with applicable laws, regulations, policies, and the organization's code of conduct.

PROCEDURES

The Committee will:

- Be composed of three to five board members

- Have no member who is an officer or employee of the organization, its subsidiaries, or its affiliates

- Be independent of management and free of any relationship that would interfere with the exercise of independent judgment as a committee member

- Have the authority to engage independent counsel and other advisors as it determines necessary to carry out its duties

- Meet in advance of meetings of the board, at least four times annually and more frequently as necessary, and make recommendations to the board annually, after consultation with the CEO, on those findings and matters within the scope of its responsibility

- Maintain minutes of all its meetings to document its activities and recommendations

- Meet periodically with the compliance officer, internal auditor, and the independent auditors to be kept informed of their independent evaluation of compliance with legal, regulatory, financial, accounting, and auditing practices

- Provide oversight for the compliance program, ensure adherence to the organization code of conduct and governmental rules and regulations, and recommend any revisions thereto, as appropriate

- Review the activities of management and its employees in light of the code of conduct and the compliance program to ensure that policies and procedures are properly understood and followed

- Review matters pertaining to education, training, and communication in connection with the code of conduct to ensure that compliance policies and procedures are properly disseminated, understood, and followed

REFERENCES/CITATIONS

OIG Compliance Program Guidance for Hospitals. Published by the Office of Inspector General in a *Federal Register* notice, dated February 23, 1998, and Supplemental Compliance Guidance January 31, 2005 (see 70 FR 4858). Available at the OIG Web site: *http://oig.hhs.gov/authorities/docs/cpghosp.pdf.*

"Corporate Responsibility and Corporate Compliance: A Resource for Health Care Boards of Directors," published by the OIG, in conjunction with the American Health Lawyers Association.

Executive compliance committee

The OIG recommends that an executive-level committee also be established to provide oversight and empowerment to the compliance officer and assist in the implementation of the compliance program. The executive-level compliance committee is seen as providing added benefits by having the perspectives of individuals with varying responsibilities and areas of knowledge in the organization, such as operations, finance, audit, human resources, and legal, as well as those involved in operations.

In healthcare organizations, this would extend to health professionals. The compliance officer should be an integral member of the committee. All committee members should have the requisite seniority and comprehensive experience within their respective areas to recommend and implement any necessary changes to policies and procedures.

OIG recommendations state that the executive compliance committee is to be established to advise the compliance officer and assist in the implementation of the compliance program. If structured appropriately, the committee can provide the compliance officer with contacts in various parts of the institution and the names of individuals who possess subject matter expertise.

If the institution employs individuals who already have responsibility for compliance in various subject areas, such as environmental safety or risk management, these individuals would be obvious candidates for the executive compliance committee.

When developing an appropriate team of people to serve as the executive compliance committee, the entity should also consider including individuals with a variety of skills and personality traits as team members. The institution should expect its compliance committee members and compliance officer to demonstrate integrity, good judgment, assertiveness, and an approachable demeanor, while eliciting the respect and trust of employees. These interpersonal skills are as important as the professional experience of the compliance officer and each member of the compliance committee.

Once members of the executive compliance committee are selected, they need to be trained on the policies and procedures of the compliance program, as well as how to discharge their duties. In essence, they should function as an extension of the compliance officer and provide the organization with increased oversight. OIG recommendations state that the committees' functions should include:

- Analyzing the organization's business environment, the legal requirements with which it must comply, and specific risk areas

- Assessing existing policies and procedures that address these risk areas for possible incorporation into the compliance program

- Working to develop standards of conduct and policies and procedures to promote compliance with the institution's program

- Recommending and monitoring, in conjunction with the relevant departments, the development of internal systems and controls to carry out the organization's standards, policies, an procedures as part of its daily operations

- Determining the appropriate strategy/approach to promote compliance with the program and detection of any potential violations, such as through hotlines and other fraud-reporting mechanisms

- Developing a system to solicit, evaluate, and respond to complaints and problems

The executive compliance committee can also be used to address other functions as the compliance concept becomes part of the overall operating structure and daily routine. It is advisable to have a governing policy for the executive compliance committee and have it approved by the board of directors. It should include the following requirements:

1. Maintenance and improvement of the code of business ethics and compliance-related policies and procedures

2. A review of organizational activities and employees in light of the code of business ethics in order to ensure that high standards of business, legal, and personal ethics are being met

3. A review of matters relating to education, training, and communications in connection with the code of business ethics and compliance program to ensure that the policies and procedures are properly disseminated, understood, and followed

It is important that evidence of the work of the executive compliance committee appear in the written record. Minutes of the meetings should be recorded, and all reports of the compliance program should also be included in the record. There should be a direct linkage to the board of directors. It is recommended that this reporting entity be a committee that provides policy guidance to the compliance program. Its roles and responsibilities should be defined, adapted to, and implemented within the corporate structure.

The executive compliance committee should be primarily an advisory and oversight body that meets monthly in the early stages of ethics/compliance program development and quarterly or as needed thereafter. The compliance officer should be a member of this committee, and other members should include leaders from various functional areas, including, but not necessarily limited to, legal counsel, human resources, internal audit, operations, and finance. The higher ranking the members of the committee, the more credible it becomes in the eyes of the employees (and regulators). The committee should make recommendations and suggestions on policies, procedures, and practices pertaining to the compliance program.

> **Best-practice tip**
>
> Formalize the creation of an executive committee with a policy and procedures document adopted by the board of directors.

TEMPLATE 4:

EXECUTIVE COMPLIANCE COMMITTEE

DEPARTMENT:	EFFECTIVE DATE:
POLICY NUMBER:	APPROVAL DATE:
POLICY: Executive Compliance Committee Policy	APPROVED BY:
POLICY REPLACED:	NUMBER OF PAGES:

BACKGROUND

The Office of Inspector General (OIG) calls for the establishment of a compliance committee to advise the compliance officer and assist in the implementation of the compliance program. We also believe in the value of an executive-level committee to provide oversight and support for the compliance program.

To this end, we have established an executive compliance committee working with the compliance officer to provide oversight, advice, and general guidance to the board of directors, chief executive officer, president, chief operating officer, and senior management on all matters relating to corporate compliance.

PURPOSE

To provide guidance on the compliance responsibilities of the executive compliance committee.

POLICY

1. The executive compliance committee has overall responsibility for continual improvement in the performance of the compliance program, including but not limited to the ongoing evaluation of corporate values, culture, and potential areas of compliance vulnerability.

2. The executive compliance committee will report to the audit and compliance committee of the board of directors on all significant issues relating to compliance with applicable laws, regulations, policies, and the code of conduct.

3. The executive compliance committee will meet periodically with the compliance officer to receive updates on the progress on all aspects of the compliance program development.

4. The executive compliance committee will maintain minutes of its meetings and ensure that compliance decisions are implemented in a timely fashion.

5. Membership of the committee consists of the CEO as chair, COO, compliance officer, legal-counsel, chief financial officer, and others designated by the chair as needed.

PROCEDURES

The executive compliance committee, working with the compliance officer and meeting at least quarterly, will:

1. Analyze the legal and regulatory requirements with which the organization must comply, as well as analyze specific risk areas

2. Ensure development, ongoing review, and updating of the code of conduct

3. Promote development and updating of compliance policies and procedures

4. Monitor and review the compliance education and training program

5. Oversee a hotline function and other systems to solicit, evaluate, and respond to complaints, allegations, and problems without fear of retribution

6. Provide guidance to executives and managers on how to promote compliance in the work environment

7. Review the need for and oversee the development of remedial actions and program improvements designed to ensure that violations of the code of conduct are not repeated

8. Oversee uniform enforcement of infractions, and ensure that matters are correctly reported in a timely fashion to appropriate outside authorities

9. Evaluate compliance program effectiveness

REFERENCES/CITATIONS

OIG Compliance Program Guidance for Hospitals. Published by the Office of Inspector General in a *Federal Register* notice, dated February 23, 1998, and Supplemental Compliance Guidance January 31, 2005 (See 70 *FR* 4858). Available at the OIG Web site: *http://oig.hhs.gov/authorities/docs/cpghosp.pdf.*

Manager and supervisor compliance responsibilities

In addition to the board and corporate executives, individual managers and supervisors share the responsibility of promoting and fostering compliance in the workplace. As noted by the OIG, compliance programs should require that promotion of, and adherence to, the elements of the compliance program be a factor in evaluating both managers' and supervisors' performance.

Managers and supervisors should be periodically trained in new compliance policies and procedures. In addition, managers and supervisors involved in the coding, claims, and cost-report development and submission processes should:

- Discuss with their employees the compliance policies and legal requirements applicable to their function

- Inform them that strict compliance with these policies and requirements is a condition of employment

- Disclose that the organization will take disciplinary action up to and including termination or revocation of privileges for violation of these policies or requirements

Template 5, *Compliance responsibilities of management*, can be found on the accompanying bonus CD-ROM (Template 2-2-5).

Template 6, *Individual employee compliance responsibilities*, can also be found on the accompanying bonus CD-ROM (Template 2-2-6).

Compliance as an element of performance

To be effective, a compliance program requires the support and participation of everyone in the work environment—executives, managers, supervisors, or employees. In recognition of this fact, the OIG encourages making the promotion of, and adherence to, the elements of the compliance program a factor in evaluating the performance of managers and supervisors. Including compliance as an element in periodic performance evaluations emphasizes the importance the organization places on compliance. This is also a best-practice tip.

This policy should also include a provision to sanction managers and supervisors if they fail to instruct their subordinates adequately, or if they fail to detect non-compliance with applicable policies and legal requirements, where reasonable diligence would have led to the discovery of problems or violations and given the organization the opportunity to correct them earlier. A sample policy, Template 7, *Compliance in performance evaluation*, is included on the accompanying CD-ROM (Template 2-2-7).

Compliance officer

The OIG guidance calls for designating a compliance officer to serve as the focal point for compliance activities. Depending on the size of the organization, this responsibility may be the individual's sole duty or added to other management responsibilities.

Providing the compliance officer with the appropriate authority is critical to the success of the program. The compliance officer should be a high-level official with direct access to the governing body and the CEO. The compliance officer should have sufficient funding and staff to perform his or her responsibilities fully.

Coordination and communication are the key functions of the compliance officer with regard to planning, implementing, and monitoring the compliance program. In a large organization, the compliance officer might be a vice president, working full-time on compliance matters. In smaller organizations, an executive's commitment might be part-time. In either case, the function should be independent and objective. Independence will help to ensure that the compliance program will be effective.

Best-practice tip

The compliance officier should be a vice president or equivalent level to fully meet the criteria suggested by the OIG.

The compliance officer's primary responsibility is to oversee and monitor implementation of the compliance program. This includes reporting on a regular basis to the board, CEO, and compliance committee on the progress of the compliance program implementation.

The compliance officer should periodically revise the program in light of changes in the needs of the organization and in the law and policies and procedures of government and private-payer health plans.

According to the OIG, the compliance officer's primary responsibilities should include, among other things:

- Overseeing and monitoring the implementation of the compliance program

- Keeping the board, CEO, and compliance committee up to date on compliance issues

- Assisting in improving efficiency and quality of services

- Reducing organization vulnerability to fraud, abuse, and waste

- Periodically revising and updating the compliance program

- Developing and coordinating compliance education/training programs

- Ensuring that contractors and agents are aware of the compliance program

- Ensuring that physicians are screened against the National Practitioner Data Bank

- Ensuring screening with the List of Excluded Individuals and Entities

- Assisting internal compliance reviews and monitoring activities

- Investigating and acting on matters related to compliance

- Taking corrective action when compliance problems have been identified

- Encouraging reporting of fraud and improprieties without fear of retaliation

The compliance officer must be given the authority to carry out these responsibilities. This includes being able review all documents and other information relevant to compliance activities, including but not limited to patient records, billing records, and records concerning the marketing efforts of the facility and the hospital's arrangements with other parties, including employees, professionals on staff, independent contractors, suppliers, agents, hospital-based physicians, etc.

This policy enables the compliance officer to review contracts and obligations (seeking the advice of legal counsel, where appropriate) that may contain referral and payment issues that could violate the Anti-kickback Statute, as well as the physician self-referral prohibition and other legal or regulatory requirements.

Inherent in the duties of the compliance officer is ensuring that all affected employees, contractors, and agents of the organization are made aware of the requirements of the compliance program through compliance education and training programs. The compliance officer must be able to coordinate with human resources, legal counsel, and financial management in coordinating internal compliance review and monitoring activities.

Best-practice tip

Establish the compliance officer function through a written charter or policy document that details his or her duties, responsibilities, and reporting obligations, and have it approved by the board.

TEMPLATE 8:

COMPLIANCE OFFICER POLICY

DEPARTMENT: COMPLIANCE OFFICE	EFFECTIVE DATE:
POLICY NUMBER:	APPROVAL DATE:
POLICY: Compliance Officer Policy	APPROVED BY:

BACKGROUND

Both the Federal Sentencing Commission and OIG Guidelines call for an executive-level compliance officer to develop, manage, and enhance the compliance program.

PURPOSE

To create a compliance officer to serve as the focal point for compliance activities and be responsible for oversight of the development, implementation, and daily operation of the compliance program.

POLICY

1. The compliance officer's primary responsibility is the design, implementation, and effective operation of the compliance program.

2. In carrying out the policy and responsibilities of the office, the compliance officer shall:

   - Have direct access to the CEO and to the board of directors

   - Not be subordinate to either the general counsel or financial officer

   - Have authority to investigate compliance violations and act as needed

   - Have access to all needed information, including contracts, billing records, and contractual arrangements

3. The executive compliance committee and the audit and compliance committee of the board of directors will provide oversight of the compliance officer's activities.

4. The compliance officer will report on a regular basis to the CEO and executive compliance committee, as well as the audit and compliance committee of the board of directors, on the progress of implementation of the compliance program.

PROCEDURES

The compliance officer will:

1. Oversee and monitor the design, implementation, and improvement of the compliance program in light of changes in the regulatory and legal environment.

2. Be responsible for developing, coordinating, and participating in a multifaceted compliance education and training program that ensures all employees and affiliated parties are educated about the code of conduct, corporate compliance program, and other specific issues deemed necessary.

3. Ensure that independent contractors and agents who furnish services are aware of the requirements of the compliance program with respect to coding, billing, and marketing, among other things.

4. Coordinate personnel issues with human resources to ensure that the List of Excluded Individuals and Entities, General Services Administration Debarment List, and National Practitioner Data Bank have been checked with respect to all employees, medical staff, and independent contractors.

5. Work with the CFO in periodic reviews, ongoing monitoring and evaluation of regulatory compliance in all business activities, and recommend development of internal systems and controls to reinforce compliance in those areas.

6. Independently investigate and act on matters related to compliance, ensuring that corrective actions are taken where compliance failures have been identified.

7. Develop and manage a hotline system and other feedback mechanisms that encourage managers and employees to report suspected fraud and other improprieties without fear of retaliation.

8. Be responsible, together with the executive compliance committee, for implementing all necessary actions to ensure achievement of the objectives of an effective compliance program by means of reviews, relevant training, a system of consistent enforcement of the rules, and the development/implementation of corrective action plans.

9. Work with the executive compliance committee in consultation with legal counsel in reviewing and updating the organization's code of conduct to ensure its continuing currency and relevance in providing guidance to management and employees.

10. Develop, maintain, and revise compliance policies and procedures for the general operation of the program and related activities to prevent illegal, unethical, or improper conduct.

11. Oversee and manage performance of the compliance program and identify potential areas of compliance vulnerability and risk. Thereafter provide specific direction as to the resolution of problematic issues, as well as general guidance on how to deal with similar situations.

12. Analyze the organization's business, industry environment, and legal requirements with which it must comply, including specific risk areas, and assess existing policies and procedures covering these areas.

13. Prepare periodic reports and evidence for the executive compliance committee and the board of directors on the progress and effectiveness of compliance activities and efforts.

14. Develop and oversee a system for uniform responses to violations of rules, regulations, policies, procedures, and the code of conduct. Where appropriate, ensure proper reporting of potential violations of law to the duly authorized law-enforcement agencies.

15. Establish audit controls and measurements to ensure correct processes are in place.

16. Maintain a working knowledge of relevant issues, laws, and regulations through periodicals, seminars, training programs, and peer contact.

17. Respond appropriately if a violation is uncovered, including a direct report to the board of directors or external agency if deemed necessary.

18. As part of ongoing auditing and monitoring, the compliance officer will arrange for an independent annual evaluation of the effectiveness of the compliance program.

REFERENCES/CITATIONS

OIG Compliance Program Guidance for Hospitals. Published by the Office of Inspector General in a *Federal Register* notice, dated February 23, 1998, and Supplemental Compliance Guidance January 31, 2005 (see 70 *FR* 4858). Available at the OIG Web site: *http://oig.hhs.gov/authorities/docs/cpghosp.pdf.*

Federal Sentencing Guidelines Manual, 2003 version can be found at *www.ussc.gov/2003guid/ TABCON03.htm.*

Compliance office and legal counsel coordination

The OIG in its Compliance Guidance stresses the importance of the chief compliance officer having the authority to review all documents and other information relevant to compliance activities, including, but not limited to:

- Patient records

- Billing records

- Records concerning the marketing efforts of the facility

- Arrangements with other parties, including:

  - Employees

  - Professionals on staff

  - Independent contractors

  - Suppliers

  - Agents

  - Organization-based physicians

This policy enables the compliance officer to review contracts and obligations (seeking the advice of legal counsel, where appropriate) that may contain referral and payment issues that could violate the Anti-Kickback Statute, as well as the physician self-referral prohibition and other legal or regulatory requirements.

The OIG also notes there is some risk to an independent compliance officer's function if it is subordinate to the legal counsel. It stresses the importance of a free-standing compliance function to ensure independent and objective legal reviews and financial analyses of the institution's compliance efforts and activities. By separating the compliance function from the legal counsel, the OIG believes a system of checks and balances is established to more effectively achieve the goals of the compliance program. Depending upon the nature of the alleged violations, an internal investigation will probably include interviews and a review of relevant documents. Some organizations should consider engaging outside counsel, auditors, or healthcare experts to assist in an investigation. Advice from in-house counsel or an outside law firm may be sought to determine the extent of liability and to plan the appropriate course of action.

The compliance officer, under advice of counsel and with guidance from governmental authorities, could be requested to continue the investigation of the reported violation. Once the investigation is completed, the compliance officer should be required to notify the appropriate governmental authority of the outcome of the investigation, including a description of the impact of the alleged violation on the operation of the applicable healthcare programs or their beneficiaries. If the investigation ultimately reveals that criminal or civil violations have occurred, the appropriate federal and state officials should be notified immediately.

The OIG recognizes that assertions of fraud and abuse by employees who may have participated in illegal conduct or committed other malfeasance raise numerous complex legal and management issues that should be examined on a case-by-case basis. The compliance officer should work closely with legal counsel, who can provide guidance regarding such issues.

Depending upon the nature of the alleged violations, an internal investigation will probably include interviews and a review of relevant documents. Some organizations should consider engaging outside counsel, auditors, or healthcare experts to assist in an investigation. A sample policy, Template 9, *Compliance office/legal counsel protocol and procedures,* is available on the bonus CD-ROM (Template 2-2-9).

Chief compliance officer and human resources management protocols

The relationship between the compliance office and human resource management should be established through a formal structure and process. Many issues raised to the compliance office directly, or through the hotline may relate to management practices that fall are the responsibility of human resources. Many issues may overlap between the compliance office and human resources.

Other issues may fall squarely in the province of human resources. However the fact that a complainant used the confidential hotline, rather than going through human resources, means the compliance officer must ensure that the promises offered through this communications channel are honored. In addition, there may be calls that include complaints or allegations against human resources.

It is therefore advisable to work out the collaboration ground rules between the compliance office and human resources in advance of any issue. This may reduce the likelihood of contentious relations, if not reduce the probability of turf fights.

The policy included on the bonus CD-ROM, Template 10, *Compliance office and human resource management protocols,* (Template 2-2-10), is drafted to create a clear distinction between the compliance office and human resources. It outlines the procedures for involving human resources in matters raised through the compliance program. By following the protocol in the policy, the organization will be in a better position to avoid confusion and/or unnecessary conflict.

Compliance officer position description

For a compliance program to work and to be perceived to be working, management has to support it, both verbally and substantively. A written policy and procedures document is a critical part of this process, but the selection of the right person for the job is also very important.

Appointing that individual as compliance officer provides tangible evidence of the organization's support for its compliance program. Providing the compliance officer the authority to oversee the development and management of the compliance program, including ensuring that it remains current with new laws and regulations, makes the decision as to who to entrust with all this power important.

An organization's size and complexity will have an effect on the selection of the compliance officer, with large organizations often designating a compliance officer. The compliance officer should have direct access to the highest levels of management and should *not* be required to report through any formal chain of command.

The compliance officer should not be identified as part of the general counsel, internal audit, or human resources. Each of these functions connotes special meaning to the employees and regulators and would not be conducive to a credible program.

Before establishing the compliance office position and appointing a compliance officer, the individual duties and responsibilities for the position should be identified. This in turn should be used in the selection criteria.

Best-practice tip

Before deciding on who should be the compliance officer, define the duties and responsibilities of the position; and those attributes, qualifications, levels of knowledge, skills, and abilities desired in the individual to be selected.

Since a compliance officer will be called upon to engage in a wide variety of activities, finding someone with the right combination of skills, experience, and judgment is critical to the success of the compliance program. There is no single background or profession for this kind of position. Successful compliance officers come from a variety of backgrounds, including legal, nursing, claims processing management, auditing, administration, and others. In fact, experience in the healthcare arena is more important than in any particular profession.

Organizations should develop a policy or position description that empowers the compliance officer position and describes its roles and responsibilities. A sample *Compliance officer position description* included on the accompanying CD-ROM provides more details concerning what a typical compliance officer position description might include.

Desired abilities for a compliance officer

The following lists should help in making determinations about the selection of the compliance officer:

- Makes sound decisions
- Operates under pressure
- Instills management confidence
- Is tenacious in resolving difficult problems
- Has a cooperative spirit in working with others in resolving problems
- Assembles the right information to fully understand problems
- Possesses the analytical skills to review documents to identify problems
- Recognizes indications of more-significant problems
- Draws conclusions by relating information from different sources
- Relates to senior management on difficult and complex issues

---

Compliance records management

According to the OIG, compliance programs should provide for the implementation of a records system that establishes policies and procedures for the creation, distribution, retention, storage, retrieval, and destruction of documents. The proper management of compliance office records is the responsibility of the compliance officer. There are a number of objectives associated with establishing a proper records-management system, including:

- Protecting the integrity of the compliance process by documenting the steps followed in identifying and resolving compliance problems.

- Providing evidence of proper management and effectiveness of the compliance program (e.g., documentation that employees were adequately trained; reports from the hotline, including the nature and results of any investigation that was conducted; modifications to the compliance program; self-disclosures; and the results of the auditing and monitoring efforts).

- Protecting the anonymity and/or confidentiality of individuals reporting suspected fraud, abuse, or other wrongdoing.

The creation and retention of such documents and reports may raise a variety of legal issues, such as patient or employee privacy and confidentiality. Therefore, as records-management policies and procedures are developed, these issues should be discussed with legal counsel.

Another purpose is to ensure that other organizational records are maintained according to policy. For example, patient medical records, billing information, and cost reports are areas that should be guided by clear records-management policies and procedures. These policies are often controlled by specific laws and regulations and, therefore, would probably be developed by legal counsel.

However, once policies are established, the compliance office may become involved in auditing and monitoring them, because they are related to compliance in many ways. For example, upon request, an organization should be able to provide documentation, such as patients' medical records and physicians' orders, to support the medical necessity of a service the organization has provided. The compliance officer should ensure that a clear, comprehensive summary of the "medical necessity" definitions and rules of the various government and private plans is prepared and disseminated appropriately.

The compliance officer must have the authority to review all documents and other information relevant to compliance activities, including, but not limited to, patient records, billing records, and records concerning the marketing efforts of the facility and the organization's arrangements with other parties, including employees, professionals on staff, independent contractors, suppliers, agents, and physicians.

This policy enables the compliance officer to review contracts and obligations (seeking the advice of legal counsel, where appropriate) that may contain referral and payment issues that could violate the Anti-Kickback Statute, as well as the physician self-referral prohibition and other legal or regulatory requirements.

Matters reported through the hotline or other communication sources that suggest substantial violations of compliance policies, regulations, or statutes should be documented and investigated promptly to determine their veracity. This includes records of receipt, retention, and treatment of complaints received regarding accounting, internal accounting controls, or auditing matters.

The compliance officer should maintain a log that records such calls, including the nature of any investigation and its results. Such information should be included in reports to the governing body, the CEO, and the compliance committee. Further, while the organization should always strive to maintain the confidentiality of an employee's identity, it should also explicitly communicate that there may be a point where the individual's identity may become known or may have to be revealed in certain instances when governmental authorities become involved.

Best-practice tip

Establish a records-management policy for the various types of compliance office records that address both retention and disposal.

Compliance office confidentiality agreement

It is essential that all people associated with the compliance office understand their special fiduciary responsibilities. These individuals will have access to confidential, proprietary, and legally privileged information. Furthermore, employees reporting problems or concerns to the compliance office may request confidentiality. Also, situations have occurred in which difficulties arose between a compliance officer and their organization.

In these situations, the organization regretted not having confidentiality agreements with the compliance officer. Therefore, a policy of confidentiality will reinforce the obligation of the compliance officer and others associated with the compliance office to keep all compliance office information secure.

A suggested confidentiality agreement is included on the accompanying bonus CD-ROM (Template 2-2-12). A template to handle confidentiality of records and policies related to recordkeeping are also included on the CD-ROM Template 13, *Compliance office non-disclosure agreement* (Template 2-2-13), and Template 14, *Compliance office records management* (Template 2-2-14).

Confidentiality and anonymity

In November 1991, the United States Sentencing Commission's "Guidelines for Organizations and Entities" called for processes to report potential violations of law. This advice translates into setting up a hotline where employees can report such conduct while protecting their anonymity and/or confidentiality up to the limits imposed by law. The hotline is a common feature in corporate compliance.

The OIG in its Compliance Guidance stresses the importance of maintaining an open line of communication between the compliance officer and employees. It is viewed as a critical element of any effective compliance program. Written policies should be developed and distributed to all employees to encourage communication and the reporting of incidents of potential fraud.

The OIG encourages the establishment of a procedure that permits employees to report matters on an anonymous basis, as well as protecting the confidentiality of those who do identify themselves but desire not to have it known that they have reported a matter to the compliance office or hotline. The compliance hotline should be implemented to address employee concerns about violations of laws, regulations, and corporate policies. Any employee who has concerns about violations of the code of conduct, policies and procedures, or unethical or suspected unlawful practices that cannot be resolved through the normal management chain should call the hotline.

Callers contacting the hotline should not be required to identify themselves. If callers identify themselves, the call should be treated confidentially and the caller's identity should be protected to the extent of the law. Introducing employees to the hotline and to the non-retaliation/non-retribution policy will also be a major component of this training.

A critical aspect of any compliance program is the establishment of a culture that encourages employees to report matters of concern on an anonymous basis, as well as protecting the confidentiality of those who do identify themselves but desire not to have it known that they have reported a matter to the compliance office or hotline.

Best-practice tip

Be aware that once there is a commitment to anonymity to callers, you must not do anything that would permit you to identify them. This means:

- No caller identification
- No record of source of incoming calls in phone invoices
- No recording of callers in voice mail

Best-practice tip

Establish a formal policy that allows employees to report problems, concerns, and potential violations anonymously or in confidence.

Related policy

Many organizations feel that they cannot fully evaluate the validity of information received without knowing the identity and position of the caller. However, weighed against this is the strong guidance by the OIG, the Sentencing Commission, and other like bodies that call for permitting anonymity.

Another factor against having callers identify themselves is that once it is done, the organization bears the obligation of protecting them against retaliation or retribution. This can become complicated and burdensome. By not knowing the identity of a caller, there is no obligation to protect them. However, anonymity offers a number of sensitive issues requiring written direction and guidance.

TEMPLATE 15:

EMPLOYEE ANONYMITY/CONFIDENTIALITY

DEPARTMENT: COMPLIANCE OFFICE	EFFECTIVE DATE:
POLICY NUMBER:	APPROVAL DATE:
POLICY: Employee Anonymity/Confidentiality	APPROVED BY: COMPLIANCE COMMITTEE
POLICY REPLACED:	NUMBER OF PAGES:

BACKGROUND

A critical aspect of an organization's compliance program is the establishment of a culture that promotes prevention, detection, and resolution of instances of conduct that do not conform to federal and state requirements, as well as the code of conduct and compliance policies.

The OIG encourages the establishment of a procedure whereby employees can report matters on an anonymous basis, while protecting the confidentiality of those who do identify themselves but desire not to have it known that they have reported a matter to the compliance office or hotline.

This policy is designed to promote this culture by enabling employees to report anonymously or in confidence problems, concerns, and potential violations of federal, state and local laws, regulations, the code of conduct, and policies and procedures by contacting the compliance office directly or through the hotline.

PURPOSE

To protect the identity of individuals who report potential compliance violations through the hotline or directly to the compliance office.

POLICY

1. All employees are responsible for reporting misconduct, including actual or potential violations of law, regulation, policy, procedure, or the code of conduct, and a telephone hotline has been established to report problems and concerns either anonymously or in confidence (see Hotline Policy).

2. Employees who report problems and concerns via the hotline in good faith will be protected from any form of retaliation or retribution (see Non-retaliation/Non-retribution Policy).

3. Everyone who receives or is assigned responsibility for hotline calls from employees shall agree to the terms of confidentiality (see Compliance Office Confidentiality Agreement Policy).

4. Employees cannot exempt themselves from the consequences of their own misconduct by reporting the issue, although self-reporting may be taken into account in determining the appropriate course of action.

5. Callers may remain anonymous, and if they identify themselves they will have their confidentiality protected to the limit of the law.

PROCEDURES

1. Anyone with knowledge of a potential violation of law, regulation, the code of conduct, policy or procedure has an affirmative duty to report that information to the compliance officer. Failure to report a potential violation may result in appropriate disciplinary action.

2. Reporting anonymously to the compliance officer can be done directly to the compliance office or by calling the hotline 24 hours a day, 365 days a year.

3. No attempt will be made to identify callers who request anonymity. When they disclose their identity, it will be held in confidence to the fullest extent practical or allowed by law.

4. Any violation of this policy may result in sanctions and penalties.

5. Determinations as to the limit of confidentiality under the law will be made in consultation with legal counsel.

REFERENCES/CITATIONS

OIG Compliance Program Guidance for Hospitals. Published by the Office of Inspector General in a *Federal Register* notice, dated February 23, 1998, and Supplemental Compliance Guidance January 31, 2005 (see 70 FR 4858). Available at the OIG Web site: *http://oig.hhs.gov/authorities/docs/cpghosp.pdf*. 2006 Federal Sentencing Guidelines Manual, Chapter 8, § 8B2.1 "Effective Compliance and Ethics Program." *www.ussc.gov/2006guid/8b2_1.html*.

Compliance Element 3: Compliance education and training

According to the OIG, one of the seven essential elements for an effective compliance program is the development and implementation of regular, effective education and training programs for all affected employees. All employees should receive training on the organization's overall compliance program.

This primary compliance training should introduce the basic aspects of the compliance program, including:

1. Compliance officer responsibilities

2. Code of conduct

3. Employee hotline

4. Problem resolution process

5. Compliance policies

Through the various compliance guidance documents, the OIG has attempted to provide a foundation for the process necessary to develop an effective and cost-efficient compliance program. The OIG recognizes that each program must be tailored to fit the needs and resources of an individual organization, depending upon its particular corporate structure, mission, and employee composition.

The statutes, regulations and guidelines of the federal and state health insurance programs, as well as the policies and procedures of the private health plans, should be integrated into every compliance training program.

The compliance officer must take steps to effectively communicate the organization's code of conduct and compliance procedures to all affected employees, physicians, independent contractors, and other significant agents. This can be done by requiring participation in training programs and disseminating publications that explain specific requirements in a practical way.

Managers of specific departments or groups can assist in identifying areas that require training and in carrying out such training. Training instructors may come from outside or inside the organization. New employees should be targeted for training early in their employment.

The OIG recommends that attendance and participation in training programs be made a condition of continued employment and that failure to comply with training requirements should result in disciplinary action. Adherence to the provisions of the compliance program, such as training requirements, should be a factor in the annual evaluation of each employee. The compliance program should retain adequate records of its training of employees, including attendance logs and material distributed at training sessions.

Compliance training should be ongoing and, at a minimum, incorporated into the orientation process. This is particularly important in organizations with high employee turnover. Periodic training updates are considered a critical element of any effective compliance program. The OIG also recommends compliance programs address the need for periodic professional education courses that may be required by statute and regulation for certain personnel.

There is little specific guidance as to the duration of the compliance training for an individual. However, it is recommended that initial compliance training for all employees be sufficient to ensure that employees understand all aspects of the compliance program.

Currently, the OIG is monitoring approximately 500 Corporate Integrity Agreements that require many of these training elements. The OIG generally requires between one and three hours annually for basic training in compliance areas. Additional training should be required for specialty fields such as billing and coding.

> **Best-practice tip**
> Provide two hours of training per employee in the first year as part of introducing the program, guidance, high-risk areas, etc. Annual training thereafter should be at least one hour in duration.

There is little guidance as to the recommended or best method for delivering compliance training, and the OIG acknowledges that a variety of teaching methods can be used effectively. Beyond that, it is up to the individual compliance program to develop effective training and education programs.

From experience, the lecture approach has been shown to be the least effective method and should be avoided. People involved in healthcare do not react well to someone lecturing to them on proper behavior and conduct in the work place. "Talking-head" videos also have limited value. Their value is primarily as part of a basic orientation or introduction to compliance training, especially when the CEO has a personal message as part of it. When that is done, the video is best limited to 8–12 minutes.

The most effective approach involves a two-tier live presentation by a facilitator. The first part of the program is delivering background information on why and how the organization has proceeded in developing a compliance program. Part of that message must cover why the program is good for employees and management alike. The facilitator should then continue to lay the ground rules of the compliance program, including going over the development and content of the standards of conduct.

The second half of the program should be devoted to taking recognizable situations and developing them into scenarios or case studies where participants can apply the standards of conduct to resolve questionable issues and determine the best way to report suspected problems. This interactive training is highly effective if a highly trained and skilled facilitator delivers it. In the hands of someone not properly prepared or equipped for the program, however it can have negative consequences.

The proper education and training of corporate officers, managers, employees, physicians, and other healthcare professionals, and the continual retraining of current personnel at all levels, are also significant elements of an effective compliance program. As part of compliance programs, organizations should require personnel to attend specific compliance training on a periodic basis.

The training should cover federal and state statutes, regulations, guidelines, the policies of private payers, and training in corporate ethics, which emphasizes the organization's commitment to compliance with these legal requirements and policies. These training programs should include sessions highlighting the organization's compliance program, summarizing fraud and abuse laws, coding requirements, claims development and submission processes, and marketing practices that reflect current legal and program standards.

An open line of communication between the compliance officer and personnel is equally important to the successful implementation of a compliance program and the reduction of any potential for fraud, abuse, and waste. Written confidentiality and non-retaliation policies should be developed and distributed to all employees during compliance training, to encourage communication and the reporting of incidents of potential fraud.

Compliance training should stress that all employees have an affirmative duty to report misconduct or violations of law, regulations, or the code of conduct. The compliance program also should develop several independent reporting paths for employees to report fraud, waste, or abuse so that they cannot be diverted by supervisors or other personnel.

The OIG encourages the use of hotlines (including anonymous hotlines), and the telephone number should be made readily available to all employees and independent contractors, possibly by conspicuously posting the telephone number in common work areas. Employees should be permitted to report matters on an anonymous basis.

Where feasible, the OIG believes that outside contractors, including physician corporations, should be afforded the opportunity to participate in or develop their own compliance training and educational programs, which complement the standards of conduct, compliance requirements, and other rules and regulations.

The OIG management advisory reports, special fraud alerts, audit and inspection reports, and advisory opinions, as well as the annual OIG *Work Plan*, are readily available from the OIG and could be the basis for the development of educational courses and programs for appropriate employees.

The compliance officer should provide direct oversight for the primary training and assistance on specialized training. (Specialized training should be developed and conducted by the appropriate management or supervisory team). The compliance officer's primary responsibilities should include developing, coordinating, and participating in a multifaceted educational and training program that focuses on the elements of the compliance program.

Furthermore, the compliance officer should ensure that all appropriate employees and management have knowledge of and comply with pertinent federal and state standards. This policy is designed to reflect the compliance officer's responsibilities related to both primary and specialized compliance training.

TEMPLATE 16:

COMPLIANCE EDUCATION AND TRAINING

DEPARTMENT: COMPLIANCE OFFICE	EFFECTIVE DATE:
POLICY NUMBER:	APPROVAL DATE:
POLICY: Compliance Education and Training	APPROVED BY:
POLICY REPLACED:	

BACKGROUND

The United States Sentencing "Guidelines for Organizations" make it manifestly clear that a compliance program must include providing employees adequate guidance as to what is expected of them in the work place.

The OIG in its Compliance Guidance underscored the critical importance of providing direction to employees on how to comply with applicable laws and regulations. The OIG notes that proper education and training of corporate officers, managers, employees, physicians, and other healthcare professionals, and the continual retraining of current personnel at all levels, are significant elements of an effective compliance program.

This policy is designed to ensure that all employees and other affected parties are made aware of their responsibility to comply with all applicable laws, regulations, compliance policies, and the code of conduct.

PURPOSE

To formalize requirements for periodic compliance education and training by all organization employees.

POLICY

1. All employees, managers, supervisors, and executives are required to attend compliance training focused on compliance with federal and state statutes, regulations, and guidelines, as well as our compliance policies, procedures, and code of conduct.

2. All training will be documented and the records maintained pursuant to our compliance records-management policy.

3. Compliance training will explain the organization, mission, and operation of the compliance program and how the compliance office operates.

4. Employees shall receive compliance education and training within 90 days of hiring.

5. Annual compliance training of one to two hours is mandatory for all employees from the executive leadership down through the various layers of the organization.

6. The compliance officer will report periodically to the executive compliance committee on the results of the compliance training program.

PROCEDURES

1. The compliance officer will develop, monitor, and ensure that compliance training and orientation meets the policy standards on this subject.

Training will:

- Explain to employees:

- Why they are undergoing training

- Why a compliance program was established

- Why compliance is in their own best interest

- How the compliance program is structured and will operate

- Introduce the compliance officer

- Include compliance policies and procedures, as well as a detailed review of all the key points of the code of conduct

- Cover how to apply the code of conduct and compliance policies to everyday work situations

- Explain that employees can report problems without fear of retribution or retaliation (see *Non-Retribution Policy*, Template 19 0n the CD-ROM Template 2-4-19)

- Ensure that employees understand how to report outside of the chain-of-command, if they believe it is necessary to do so using their employee hotline

- Emphasize to employees the ability to report concerns, allegations, and suspected wrong-doing anonymously or, if they do identify themselves, assure them of confidentiality, to the limit of the law

Compliance trainers must be knowledgeable of:

- The compliance program

- Applicable federal laws and regulations

- Requirements of the Sentencing Commission Guidelines

- Relevant policies and procedures

- The operations of the compliance program

- The content of the code of conduct

2. Sign-in sheets will be used in all training sessions to document employees' reception of compliance training, and everyone undergoing training must sign in at the time they receive their training.

3. All participants in compliance training will receive a copy of the code of conduct for use during the class.

4. Once employees have signed in for training, they cannot leave the session without it being reflected on the sign-in log.

5. Training protocols and materials must be standardized, so as to provide evidence that anyone who signed in for training will have received the same instruction.

6. It is very important to document that employees were given the opportunity to question and apply the principles of the code of conduct to various workplace situations.

7. Evaluation forms will be used after every compliance training class to measure the effectiveness of the training sessions. Participants in each training session will be asked to complete a short evaluation of the program that will be collected directly by someone in the compliance office. The compliance officer will maintain the evaluation forms in order to monitor the quality and effectiveness of the training.

REFERENCES/CITATIONS

OIG Compliance Program Guidance for Hospitals. Published by the Office of Inspector General in a *Federal Register* notice, dated February 23, 1998, and Supplemental Compliance Guidance January 31, 2005 (see 70 *FR* 4858). Available at the OIG Web site: *http://oig.hhs.gov/authorities/docs/cpghosp.pdf.*

"Corporate Responsibility and Corporate Compliance: A Resource for Health Care Boards of Directors," published by the OIG, in conjunction with the American Health Lawyers Association.

Compliance Element 4: Hotline to receive complaints

The OIG believes that whistleblowers should be protected against retaliation, a concept embodied in the provisions of the False Claims Act. Employees or former employees sometimes sue their employers under the False Claims Act's qui tam provisions out of frustration because the organization has failed to act when a questionable, fraudulent, or abusive situation was brought to the attention of senior corporate officials. Therefore, the organization should adopt a strict non-retaliation policy to support its open communication policy.

It is clear that organizations need to have a reporting mechanism outside the "chain of command." This translates to an employee hotline. The hotline has existed for decades in some form but did not become common until relatively recently. As noted in the previous section, consideration for using the hotline as a compliance program tool got a boost in the defense industry as result of the Department of Justice crackdowns on contractor frauds.

Most settlements and agreements between contractors and the federal government have included a provision for the establishment of a hotline. During the same period of time, all the Offices of Inspector General of the federal government, along with the General Accounting Office, initiated similar programs. As scandals spread to other industries, so did the popularity of hotlines as a corrective action measure. In June 1992, the United States Sentencing Commission "Guidelines for Organizations" went into effect, all but mandating the establishment of hotlines.

The OIG says the creation of a hotline to receive complaints is one of the seven essential elements of an effective compliance program. In establishing the hotline, it is critical to create and maintain a system of procedures that protect complainants and whistleblowers from identification and retaliation. The OIG encourages the use of anonymous hotlines, e-mails, written memoranda, newsletters, and other forms of information exchange to maintain open lines of communication.

A good starting point for establishing a hotline function is through the chartering process. Depending on the number of people managing the compliance program, there may be a designated individual responsible for the hotline function. If so, that function should be defined and chartered as part of the compliance office operation.

This document can be used to lay the issues before management and define exactly what is to be done in developing a hotline operation. Once a charter has been approved at the executive and board level of the organization, a more definitive policy and procedures document can define how it will operate in practice. A sample charter, Template 17, *Hotline charter,* has been included on the accompanying CD-ROM (Template 2-4-17).

The OIG recognizes that assertions of fraud and abuse by employees who may have participated in illegal conduct or committed other malfeasance raise complex legal and management issues that should be examined on a case-by-case basis. The compliance officer should work closely with legal counsel in developing written guidance regarding such issues.

Make sure that your hotline policy:

- Includes calls for queries, complaints, and allegations of wrongdoing

- Ensures anonymity and confidentiality

- Balances the rights of the accuser and the accused

- Maintains proper records of calls and actions taken

- Follows the appropriate investigative protocols

- Protects against retaliation and retribution

- Documents proper operation of the program

- Provides feedback to employees and management

- Reports results to the executive level

- Follows records-management retention and destruction policies

A number of very sensitive and complex concerns for compliance officers and committees to consider include:

- Who should be responsible for the hotline function

- How the call should be answered, and by whom

- Hours of operation

- The kind of training the individuals answering the call should have

Making mistakes on these decisions can be very costly. A botched call may result in serious liabilities to the organization, as well as loss of confidence by employees in the hotline as a means of communication. The alternatives for them could be reporting the matter to a government agency, newspaper, or attorney. None of these would be very appealing to organization management, which would have to deal with the consequences of such actions. The easiest solutions to these problems are included in the following best-practice tips.

Best-practice tip
- Use a toll-free number
- Hotline should optimally be available whenever a caller feels the need to make a call (24 hours a day, 365 days)
- Hotline should permit anonymity to callers
- Confidentiality must be protected when asked for
- Those taking calls should be thoroughly trained on the issues likely to be raised by callers

---

Among the more difficult decisions is the question of who should be taking the calls. Remember, these hotline calls may be of an extremely sensitive nature. Many calls will provide extremely complicated facts that command the complete attention of the individual taking the call. Those charged with taking calls must be trained on debriefing techniques, compliance issues, and how to avoid being entrapped by callers.

Some considerations on this and other questions revolve around the most important decision: Should the hotline be operated in-house, or should it be contracted out to a service? In making the decision, consider the following factors:

- The number of hotline calls annually will approximate 1%–2% of the employee population. Divide that number by 12 for the estimated calls per month. Those calls will not be distributed evenly over the month.

- Someone should be available to take a call during all working hours, preferably 24/7. The problem that is you cannot predict when the phone will ring. However, rest assured that the most important hotline call will be received when the operator is away from his or her post.

- It takes time to gain necessary rapport with callers before full debriefing can take place. Hotline operators must project patience, empathy and caring. Unfortunately, callers may not get right to the point and identify their problem or issue. Employees calling in are often nervous and unsure that they really want to be making the call, and most are genuinely fearful of the ramifications of their call. This is true even after assurances by their company of non-retaliation and anonymity.

- Only highly trained hotline specialists should be used to establish necessary rapport, properly debrief, and channel the information correctly, in a form that is understandable and actionable. This requires a dedicated staff.

- Hotline operators require privacy, and they should have their own space where it is quiet. A hotline call can take two minutes or two hours—you never know until you are in the middle of one. The operator cannot be interrupted in the middle of the call and certainly should not end the call until the caller is finished.

- At a minimum, a company answering its own hotline will require at least 1.5 staff-years just to staff the phones during a normal eight-hour period. After all, the operator will sometimes go to lunch, to the restroom, and on vacation (where there are no phones). Assuming one staff-year costs $30,000, labor alone will total approximately $45,000. Divide the expected number of calls in a year into that number to approximate the cost per call. On top of that, you must add the cost of the telephone line, the cost of the space, and the cost of training and re-training operators. For example, a company with 2,000 employees may expect 20 to 40 calls per year or a rough average of one call per week. The estimated cost per call would run about $1,500 to $2,250—the larger the employee base, the less the cost per call.

- Comparing the estimated cost of operating an internal hotline with the cost to engage companies that specialize in outsourcing the service clearly demonstrates that outsourcing this service is usually considerably less expensive than operating a hotline in-house.

- Hotline service companies have personnel who are experienced and trained in answering hotline calls. That is all they do—they are specialists and may be better prepared to spot hidden problems or issues.

- Staff members may be more comfortable talking with someone "on the outside." They recognize that there is very little likelihood they will be recognized. Studies have shown that employees are more likely to discuss a highly sensitive issue with someone outside the company than with a company employee.

- Reputable hotline service companies are in a position to recognize issues of sensitive regulatory or enforcement significance. Many companies provide trending and tracking information that can be used for periodic reporting to executive leadership regarding the hotline operations.

Best-practice tip

The most effective hotlines are those operated by professionals. Consider first using vendors operating under protocols and written instructions, rather than operating a hotline in-house. Costs are negligible in comparison to trying to operate one in-house.

If a decision is made to outsource the answering of the compliance hotline, using only a service that has live operators taking the calls is very important for many reasons, such as:

- Having voice mail or recorded, messaging is not efficient, and it may cause a lot of problems.

Recording a voice may violate a commitment to protect anonymity (see Anonymity Policy template). If the voice is recorded, it might lead to the identity of the caller.

- There is a heightened concern about privacy in the country today. Many states have enacted laws for protecting privacy. Some state laws may create problems for those recording a caller's voice.

- Another important point is that studies have shown that people calling a hotline will not want to (nor will they) leave sensitive information. This deters callers or invites them to go elsewhere with their concerns, allegations, and information. If they do leave information of interest, there will be no way to fully debrief them, and chances are that a lot of vital information will not be included in the recording.

- If a recording of calls is known, those recordings may be subpoenaed or otherwise ordered into a court case as part of a wrongful discharge suit, class-action case, investigation, etc.

- Never use a service that includes recording of the caller's voice. It can be a costly mistake.

- There are a variety of services offered by most hotline vendors and many whistles and bells to differentiate them. Each may have something they consider to be a unique feature of possible use by a client. However, the following are some critical factors that should be considered in selecting a hotline vendor:

    1. **Test call the vendor.** Never buy a "pig in a poke." Every hotline vendor should permit anonymous "test calls" by prospective clients. A prospective client should be able to call in to provide a fictitious report without the operator knowing it is a test call. The operator should not be able to know it is a test call because it is coming in on an active shared toll-free hotline number. By this means, the prospective client can determine the amount of time it took for the hotline service to answer the call, the debriefing skills of the operator in obtaining all the relevant facts, and the quality and accuracy of the call report results.

    2. **Ensure the vendor has back-up power.** Never trust your hotline to a vendor that cannot guarantee service under all circumstances. There have been a number of examples of power outages around the country in recent years. Some of these outages after a hur-

ricane or tornado have caused blackouts for whole regions for many days. A variation on "Murphy's Law" is that the most important hotline call the organization will ever have will be made when the party on the receiving end is least prepared to receive it. No organization should gamble that a hotline service may not be available during such an outage. A serious hotline vendor will have its own generator as part of any effective disaster recovery program. What you don't need is to have a small disaster of your own because your vendor was not able to provide the service when it was most needed.

3. **Only professionally trained/educated parties should take your calls.** Some of the most sensitive information that a company or organization may have could become part of a hotline call. What is not needed is an underpaid, undereducated, hourly worker taking the call like some answering service. Calls made on your hotline may involve complicated financial matters, regulatory issues, highly emotional or sensitive personnel issues, etc. Demand that all operators taking the calls be full-time employees (not part-time or temporary ones), college educated, and fully trained on the types of issues that could be raised on your hotline.

4. **Hotline clients should be held by service, not contract.** Look at vendor contracts carefully. There are many tricks to "lock in" clients. If a vendor insists on annual contracts that cannot be easily terminated and/or where termination procedures are complicated, then beware. Those vendors that lock in their clients with contracts rather than by good services should be suspect. Insist on being able to cancel a contract at any time without cause, with a simple written notice. If the service is good, there should be no concerns in granting this request. Similarly, if there is a client-specific call number used in the service, ensure that the number can be retained by your organization, should there be a termination of service for any reason. It is a common trick by vendors to get a client to publicize a toll-free number that they own so that canceling the contract would create a host of problems with changing to another number.

5. **Always insist on a single account representative.** Once a vendor is selected, it is important that optimum service follows. That means there should be a single point of contact with the vendor for any and all issues, whether related to the quality of the reports, changes in protocols, or an invoice. It should not be the client who has to chase down the right party to get the right action.

6. **Demand that the services meet your needs, not the other way around.** It is important to decide on exactly what is needed, how it should be delivered, and to whom. Then it is a matter of the hotline vendor meeting those criteria. This may (and should) require the vendor to customize services for the client. If a vendor insists on the organization accept-

ing the vendor's model and resists customizing, then move on to another vendor. "The customer is always right" applies here just as much as to other business sectors.

The compliance officer should document such calls by maintaining a log of all calls and the nature of each investigation. A hotline record system must be established that includes a case-number system. The data to be used to report into the system will include the date of the complaint and the nature of the problem (e.g., poor management practices, theft of property, violation of company policies, etc.). (Refer to Compliance Office Records Management Policy, Template 14 located on the CDROM Template 2-2-24). Such information should be included in reports to the governing body, the CEO, and the compliance committee. The employee hotline is an open invitation to employees to bring a wide variety of troubling issues to one focal point.

Best-practice tip

When developing a hotline policy document be very specific as to the written guidance so that everyone understands fully their obligations to report and how those reports will be handled.

TEMPLATE 18:

COMPLIANCE HOTLINE

DEPARTMENT: Compliance Office	EFFECTIVE DATE:
POLICY NUMBER:	APPROVAL DATE:
POLICY: Compliance Hotline Policy	APPROVED BY:
POLICY REPLACED:	NUMBER OF PAGES:

BACKGROUND

The OIG encourages the use of anonymous hotlines, e-mails, written memoranda, newsletters, and other forms of information exchange to maintain open lines of communication. The hotline telephone number should be made readily available to all employees and independent contractors by being conspicuously posted in common work areas.

The posting should state that an employee hotline has been established to permit a confidential process for reporting any possible or potential violation of federal, state, or local laws regulations; the code of conduct; or policies and procedures. It should then state that this hotline permits the anonymity of the reporter to be preserved.

The purpose of this hotline is to ensure the timely identification and resolution of all issues that may adversely affect employees, patients or the organization. The hotline is one of several communication channels to report problems and concerns. Employees are expected to report problems or concerns either anonymously or in confidence via the hotline when they believe a potential violation has taken place.

PURPOSE

To provide guidance on the operation of the compliance hotline

POLICY

1. All employees are responsible for reporting misconduct, including actual or potential violations of law, regulation, policy, procedure, or the code of conduct.

2. A telephone hotline permits employees to report problems and concerns anonymously. If they identify themselves, their confidentiality will be protected to the limit of the law (see Employee Anonymity/Confidentiality Policy).

3. Employees who report problems and concerns via the hotline in good faith will be protected from any form of retaliation or retribution. Any employee who commits or condones any form of retaliation will be subject to discipline up to and including termination (see Non-retaliation/Non-retribution Policy).

4. All those who are employed in the hotline operation are expected to act with utmost discretion and integrity in ensuring that information received is acted upon in a reasonable and proper manner. Everyone who receives or is assigned responsibilities for hotline calls from employees will agree to the terms of confidentiality (see Compliance Office Confidentiality Agreement Policy).

5. The compliance officer is responsible for the daily operation of the employee hotline.

6. Employees are strongly encouraged to report problems and concerns via the chain of command or human resources before resorting to the employee hotline. However, this communication channel is always available if special circumstances exist or their issue is not being properly addressed.

7. Employees cannot exempt themselves from the consequences of their own misconduct by reporting the issue, although self-reporting may be taken into account in determining the appropriate course of action.

8. The hotline will be answered by a live person who will debrief the caller and make a report on all information provided.

PROCEDURES

1. Anyone with knowledge of a potential violation of law, regulation, the code of conduct, policy, or procedure has an affirmative duty to report that information to the compliance officer. Failure to report a potential violation may result in appropriate disciplinary action.

2. Reporting anonymously to the compliance officer can be done directly by calling the hotline 24 hours a day, 365 days a year.

3. The compliance officer will log all calls made to the hotline to include the nature of the complaint or violation reported, the date and time reported, the source of the information, and the department or facility affected.

4. The compliance officer will determine what further investigation is required into the reported complaint or potential violation.

5. Disciplinary or corrective action for all substantiated allegations will be an integral part of the compliance program.

6. Knowledge of misconduct, including actual or potential violations of law, regulation, policy, procedure, or the code of conduct, must be immediately reported to management, the compliance officer, or the employee hotline.

7. Concerns regarding any issue should be addressed in the following order:

   - Immediate supervisor

   - Department manager

   - Department head/director

   - Senior administrative officer of the organization

8. The compliance officer is responsible for the hotline operation. This includes ensuring that all hotline calls are addressed in an appropriate and timely manner, as well as in accordance with these and all other related policies and procedures. Other responsibilities include:

   - Ensuring proper functioning of the hotline

   - Establishing reporting and records-maintenance procedures

   - Conducting appropriate investigations and follow-up

   - Referring calls when appropriate

   - Providing feedback to callers when necessary

   - Reporting hotline activity to the oversight committee

   - Maintaining security for all calls and related documents

9. Those who answer the hotline must be properly trained personnel.

10. All callers to the hotline will hear the same pre-recorded message explaining their rights, any limitations, non-retaliation policy, and other pertinent information. All callers will then be

given the opportunity to speak with a live operator (see Non-Retaliation Policy Template 19 on CD-ROM Template 2-4-19).

11. No attempt will be made to identify a caller who requests anonymity (see Anonymity Policy Template 15 on CD-ROM Template 2-215).

12. Whenever callers disclose their identity, it will be held in confidence to the fullest extent practical or allowed by law.

13. The compliance officer will communicate any matter deemed potentially unlawful to legal counsel.

14. Calls will be documented on the confidential hotline intake form. All call records will be logged, sequentially numbered upon receipt on this form, and placed in the care and custody of the compliance officer.

15. When a hotline call cannot be resolved while the caller is on the line, a follow-up review or investigative actions will be taken. The caller may be asked to call back at an agreed date and time in case additional information is needed. Callers will be provided an identification number to protect their identity.

16. The hotline operation will involve other departments, as appropriate, for advice or further investigation. In the event that the compliance officer is not, in good faith, satisfied that a matter brought before the aforesaid departments was appropriately addressed and resolved, the compliance officer will be responsible for and is authorized to take the matter to other persons in positions of authority.

17. The compliance officer will report periodically to the compliance committee and the board of directors regarding hotline activity. This report will include the total number of calls received and acted upon and the general results from the hotline operation. In addition, the report will include any recommendations for system-wide improvements or corrective actions arising from the results of the operation and related investigations.

18. Management must take appropriate measures to ensure support for this policy and encourage the reporting of problems and concerns. At a minimum, the following actions should be taken and become an ongoing aspect of the management process:

   • Meet with subordinates and discuss the main points within this policy

   • Provide all subordinates with a copy of this policy

   • Post a copy of this policy on employee bulletin boards

19. One of the primary responsibilities of the compliance office is to ensure that employees are allowed to report problems and concerns without fear of retaliation. Therefore, it is critical that the organization adopt a formal non-retaliation policy and that all employees are aware of and understand the policy. Any indication of a violation of the non-retaliation policy should be investigated immediately by the compliance office. Discipline should be significant if violations of the non-retaliation policy are substantiated.

REFERENCES/CITATIONS

OIG Compliance Program Guidance for Hospitals. Published by the Office of Inspector General in a *Federal Register* notice, dated February 23, 1998, and Supplemental Compliance Guidance January 31, 2005 (see 70 *FR* 4858). Available at the OIG Web site: *http://oig.hhs.gov/authorities/docs/cpghosp.pdf.*

"Corporate Responsibility and Corporate Compliance: A Resource for Health Care Boards of Directors," published by the OIG, in conjunction with the American Health Lawyers Association.

Whistleblower protection

A key element of any effective compliance program includes a prohibition on the firing, threatening, or otherwise harming any person on the basis of the employee's reporting or participating in resolving a compliance issue, especially those relating to violation of laws by the organization.

This warrant of protection is to encourage employees and others in a position to report violations of law by protecting them against retaliation. Therefore, people who bring organizational problems or criminal conduct in a company to the attention of the hotline or compliance officer may be entitled to protections and remedies, such as reinstatement, back pay, and special damages.

Best-practice tip
- Ensure that this policy is made easily available to all employees
- Include a reference to this policy in the code of conduct
- All compliance training should address this policy
- Reinforce this policy with all supervisors and managers

At a minimum, comprehensive compliance programs should contain a process, such as a hotline, to receive complaints, and the adoption of procedures to protect the anonymity of complainants and to protect whistleblowers from retaliation. The compliance officer's responsibilities include developing policies and programs that encourage managers and employees to report suspected fraud and other improprieties without fear of retaliation.

The OIG believes that whistleblowers should be protected against retaliation, a concept embodied in the provisions of the False Claims Act. In many cases, employees sue their employers under the False Claims Act's qui tam provisions out of frustration because of the employer's failure to take action when a questionable, fraudulent, or abusive situation was brought to the attention of senior corporate officials.

The OIG calls for written confidentiality and non-retaliation policies to be developed and distributed to all employees to encourage communication and the reporting of incidents of potential fraud. Without these guarantees, it is not likely that actions against those who fail to report can be sustained.

A policy document should be very specific as to what commitment and conditions the organization is defining in their warranting non-retaliation. It should also underscore the affirmative duty to report suspected wrongdoing. A sample, Template 19, *Non-retaliation policy,* is included on the bonus CD-ROM (Template 2-4-19).

Supervisor certification of briefing to employees on non-retaliation policy

Some organizations go further to reinforce the non-retaliation policy by having supervisors and managers certify they have briefed their employees on it. When doing this, it is important that protocols be established to collect and maintain these certifications as part of the compliance office records. The following template is an example of this type of form.

TEMPLATE 20:

SUPERVISOR CERTIFICATION OF BRIEFING TO EMPLOYEES ON NON-RETALIATION POLICY

This is to certify that all employees who report to me have received a copy of and have been personally briefed on the content and importance of the Non-Retaliation Compliance Policy, as well as those sections of the code of conduct relating to the treatment of employees and the creation of a work environment that promotes open communication have been reviewed with all employees.

Facility _____

Department _____

Name of Supervisor/ Manager _____

(Please print)

_____

(Signature)   (Date)

*Send completed form to the compliance officer at _____.

Compliance Element 5: Response and enforcement

An effective compliance program should include guidance regarding disciplinary action for corporate officers, managers, employees, physicians, and other healthcare professionals who have failed to comply with the organization's standards of conduct, policies and procedures, or federal and state laws. A sample policy, Template 21, *Investigation policy*, located on the accompanying CD-ROM (Template 2-5-21), outlines how an effective compliance program should conduct internal investigations once a concern is raised.

Compliance issue resolution process

According to the OIG, one of the seven essential elements for an effective compliance program is the investigation and remediation of identified systemic problems. Furthermore one of the primary responsibilities of the compliance officer is to receive and resolve compliance issues raised by employees.

The compliance office can be expected to learn of compliance issues and concerns via the employee hotline, direct contact, or auditing and monitoring. In any case, the compliance office should handle all issues consistently to ensure that the integrity of the office is maintained and that all matters receive appropriate attention.

Appropriate response to any detected offense should include the implementation of modifications to the program necessary in order to prevent future offenses of the same kind. Many compliance issues involve matters of significant legal concern. Therefore, it is necessary that the compliance officer and legal counsel (either inside or outside counsel) establish a working relationship. However, the compliance office and chief compliance officer should not be subordinate to legal as this raises questions of autonomy. Furthermore, many issues raised to the compliance office will not involve legal matters and should therefore not require legal assistance. It is noted that there are other issues wherein legal counsel is appropriate and essential. Those situations are addressed in the protocols between the compliance office and legal counsel.

The accompanying policy, Template 22, *Compliance issue resolution*, located on the bonus CD-ROM (Template 2-5-22) provides guidance for issue resolution, notwithstanding the channel through which it was raised.

Enforcement and discipline

An effective compliance program should include guidance regarding disciplinary action for corporate officers, managers, employees, physicians, and other healthcare professionals who have failed to comply with the standards of conduct, policies and procedures, or federal and state laws, or those who have otherwise engaged in wrongdoing, any of which has the potential to impair the organization's status as a reliable, honest, and trustworthy healthcare provider.

The OIG believes that the compliance program should include a written policy statement setting forth the degrees of disciplinary action that may be imposed upon corporate officers, managers, employees, physicians, and other healthcare professionals for failing to comply with the standards, policies, and applicable statutes and regulations.

Intentional or reckless non-compliance should subject transgressors to significant sanctions. Such sanctions could range from oral warnings to suspension, privilege revocation (subject to any applicable peer-review procedures), financial penalties, or termination, as appropriate.

The written standards of conduct should elaborate on the procedures for handling disciplinary problems and those who will be responsible for taking appropriate action. Some disciplinary actions can be handled by department managers, while others may have to be resolved by a senior administrator.

Disciplinary action may be appropriate where a responsible employee's failure to detect a violation is attributable to his or her negligence or reckless conduct. Personnel should be advised that disciplinary action will be taken on a fair and equitable basis. Managers and supervisors should they have a responsibility to discipline employees in an appropriate and consistent manner.

The consequences of non-compliance should be consistently applied and enforced in order for the disciplinary policy to have the required deterrent effect. All levels of employees should be subject to the same disciplinary action for the commission of similar offenses.

The commitment to compliance applies to all personnel levels within an organization. The OIG believes that corporate officers, managers, supervisors, medical staff, and other healthcare professionals should be held accountable for the actual or potential failure of their subordinates to adhere to the applicable standards, laws, and procedures. An sample policy, Template 23, *Enforcement and discipline policy,* is located on the accompanying bonus CD-ROM (Template 2-5-23).

Table of penalties

According to the OIG, an effective compliance program should include the enforcement of appropriate disciplinary action against employees who violate internal compliance policies, applicable statutes, regulations or federal healthcare program requirements.

Clearly, the federal government places a high priority on healthcare companies addressing this issue. Enforcement of appropriate disciplinary action against employees at all levels involves developing this element of a compliance program as prescribed by and consistent with the OIG *Compliance Program Guidance for Hospitals* provisions on this subject.

The OIG believes the compliance program should include a written sanction policy setting forth the degrees of disciplinary actions that may be imposed upon corporate officers, managers, employees, physicians, and other healthcare professionals for failing to comply with the organization's standards and policies, and applicable statutes and regulations. Intentional or reckless non-compliance should subject transgressors to significant sanctions.

Such sanctions could range from oral warnings to suspension, privilege revocation (subject to any applicable peer-review procedures), termination, or financial penalties, as appropriate. The written standards of conduct should elaborate both on the procedures for handling disciplinary problems and on those who will be responsible for taking appropriate action.

Some disciplinary actions can be handled by department managers, while others may have to be resolved by a senior organization administrator. Disciplinary action may be appropriate where a responsible employee's failure to detect a violation is attributable to his or her negligence or reckless conduct.

It is vital to publish and disseminate the range of disciplinary standards for improper conduct and to educate officers and other staff regarding these standards. The consequences of non-compliance should be consistently applied and enforced, in order for the disciplinary policy to have the required deterrent effect.

All levels of employees should be subject to the same disciplinary action for the commission of similar offenses. The commitment to compliance applies to all personnel levels within an organization. The OIG believes that corporate officers, managers, supervisors, medical staff, and other healthcare professionals should be held accountable for failing to comply with, or for the foreseeable failure of their subordinates to adhere to, the applicable standards, laws, and procedures.

The OIG believes that some violations may be so serious that they warrant immediate disclosure or notification to governmental authorities, prior to, or simultaneous with, commencing an internal investigation, such as, if the conduct:

- Is a clear violation of criminal law

- Has a significant adverse effect on the quality of care provided to program beneficiaries (in addition to any other legal obligations regarding quality of care)

- Indicates evidence of a systemic failure to comply with applicable laws, an existing corporate integrity agreement, or other standards of conduct, regardless of the financial impact on federal healthcare programs

The OIG calls for uniform enforcement that takes into consideration the gravity of the infraction and progressive penalties for repeat offenders. It also calls for publishing and disseminating the range of disciplinary standards for improper conduct and educating officers and other staff regarding these standards.

Although the preceding policy document may be deemed sufficient to adequately address this area, many organizations desire to go further by developing a "table of penalties" as a way to better address these standards. For those opting for this approach, it is important to provide guidance but also sufficient latitude to permit taking into consideration extenuating, mitigating, and aggravating circumstances in individual situations.

In short, the guidance should be flexible and not handcuff managers in carrying out their responsibilities. The following should guide the development of a draft table of penalties:

1. The OIG noted, "It is vital to publish and disseminate the range of disciplinary standards for improper conduct, and to educate officers and other staff regarding these standards." This requirement can be addressed through the development of a standardized table of penalties. It is also important that the underlying issue(s) leading to a penalty be included in compliance training and tracked back to the code of conduct.

2. According to the OIG, "All levels of employees should be subject to the same disciplinary action for the commission of similar offenses," and "the commitment to compliance applies to all personnel levels within an organization." A table of penalties will encourage standard disciplinary action across all levels of employees within the organization.

3. The OIG believes that "the compliance program should include a written policy statement setting forth the degrees of disciplinary actions that may be imposed upon corporate officers, managers, employees, physicians and other healthcare professionals for failing to comply with the standards and policies, and applicable statutes and regulations."

4. The OIG guidance further states, "Intentional or reckless non-compliance should subject trans-gressors to significant sanctions," and "such sanctions could range from oral warnings to sus-pension, privilege revocation (subject to any peer review procedures), termination, or financial penalties, as appropriate."

5. The table of penalties must, therefore, include graduated penalties depending on the severity of the infraction and must be progressive depending on the number of times an action occurs.

6. The reference by the OIG to compliance with "standards and policies and applicable statutes and regulations" necessitates that the table of penalties be tied to the code of conduct that is disseminated to all employees. The code of conduct should refer to the table of penalties, and it should include a statement to the effect that employees who violate the code of conduct and other established policies will be subject to appropriate actions as set forth in the table of pen-alties guidance.

7. The OIG notes that "written standards of conduct should elaborate on the procedures for han-dling disciplinary problems and those who will be responsible for taking appropriate action." The table of penalties should, therefore, describe how officials should review, evaluate, and determine the application of the penalties.

8. Another significant aspect of this effort is establishing the process for periodic reviews of dis-ciplinary actions. Such reviews will ensure fair and consistent application of the penalties outlined in the sample Table of Penalties included on this book's bonus CD-ROM (Template 2-5-24).

Best-practice tip

If a table-of-penalties approach is followed, ensure wide latitude in applying it to allow for extenuating, mitigating, and aggravating circumstances. The table should only be a guide, not a rule book.

Voluntary disclosure to third parties

The OIG currently maintains a voluntary disclosure program that encourages providers to report suspected fraud. The concept of voluntary self-disclosure is premised on recognition that the govern-ment alone cannot protect the integrity of Medicare and other federal healthcare programs. Healthcare providers must be willing to police themselves, correct underlying problems, and work with the govern-ment to resolve these matters. The OIG voluntary self-disclosure program has four prerequisites:

1. The disclosure must be on behalf of an entity, not an individual

2. The disclosure must be truly voluntary (i.e., no pending proceeding or investigation)

3. The entity must disclose the nature of the wrongdoing and the harm to the federal programs

4. The entity must not be the subject of a bankruptcy proceeding before or after the self-disclosure

Violations of a compliance program, failure to comply with applicable federal or state law, and other types of misconduct threaten an organization's status as a reliable, honest, and trustworthy provider capable of participating in federal healthcare programs. Detected but uncorrected misconduct can seriously endanger the mission, reputation, and legal status of the organization.

Consequently, upon reports or reasonable indications of suspected non-compliance, it is important that the compliance officer or other management officials initiate prompt steps to investigate the conduct in question in order to determine whether a material violation of applicable law or the requirements of the compliance program has occurred.

If so, he or she must take steps to correct the problem. As appropriate, such steps may include an immediate referral to criminal and/or civil law enforcement authorities, a corrective action plan, a report to the government, and the submission of any overpayments, if applicable.

Where potential fraud or False Claims Act liability is not involved, the OIG recognizes that CMS regulations and contractor guidelines already include procedures for returning overpayments to the government as they are discovered. However, even if the overpayment detection and return process is working and is being monitored by the organization's audit or coding divisions, the OIG still believes the compliance officer needs to be told of these overpayments, violations, or deviations, and that the officer should look for trends or patterns demonstrating a systemic problem.

Depending upon the nature of the alleged violations, an internal investigation will probably include interviews and a review of relevant documents. Some organizations should consider engaging outside counsel, auditors, or healthcare experts to assist in an investigation.

Records of the investigation should contain:

- Documentation of the alleged violation

- Description of the investigative process

- Copies of interview notes

- Key documents

- A log of witnesses interviewed and documents reviewed

- The results of the investigation (e.g., any disciplinary action taken) and the corrective action implemented

Although any action taken as the result of an investigation will necessarily vary depending upon the organization and the situation, organizations should strive for some consistency by utilizing sound practices and disciplinary protocols. Further, after a reasonable period, the compliance officer should review the circumstances that formed the basis for the investigation to determine whether similar problems have been uncovered.

According to the OIG, if an investigation of an alleged violation is undertaken and the compliance officer believes that the integrity of the investigation may be at stake because of the presence of employees under investigation, those subjects should be removed from their current work activity until the investigation is completed (unless an internal or government-led undercover operation is in effect).

In addition, the compliance officer should take appropriate steps to secure or prevent the destruction of documents or other evidence relevant to the investigation. If the organization determines that disciplinary action is warranted, it should be prompt and imposed in accordance with the organization's written standards of disciplinary action.

If the compliance officer, the compliance committee, or a management official discovers credible evidence of misconduct from any source and, after a reasonable inquiry, has reason to believe that the misconduct may violate criminal, civil, or administrative law, then the organization should promptly report the existence of misconduct to the appropriate governmental authority within a reasonable period, but not more than 60 days after determining that there is credible evidence of a violation.

Prompt reporting will demonstrate the organization's good faith and willingness to work with governmental authorities to correct and remedy the problem. In addition, reporting such conduct will be considered a mitigating factor by the OIG in determining administrative sanctions (e.g., penalties, assessments, and exclusion) if the reporting provider becomes the target of an OIG investigation.

TEMPLATE 25:

DISCLOSURE OF MISCONDUCT

DEPARTMENT: Compliance Office	EFFECTIVE DATE:
POLICY NUMBER:	APPROVAL DATE:
POLICY: Disclosure of Misconduct	APPROVED BY:
POLICY REPLACED:	NUMBER OF PAGES:

BACKGROUND

One of the primary purposes of the compliance program is to identify any misconduct that could constitute a violation of criminal, civil, or administrative law and, if found to be an actual violation, take steps to address the misconduct. As appropriate, such steps may include a voluntary disclosure to an appropriate third-party law enforcement or regulatory agency.

Detection and timely reporting of misconduct will help maintain the integrity of the organization and preserve its status as a reliable, honest, and trustworthy healthcare provider. Furthermore, penalties and sanctions can be materially reduced if an organization voluntarily discloses violations of civil, criminal, or administrative law in a timely manner.

PURPOSE

To establish a process within the structure of the corporate compliance program to address potential or actual misconduct, including voluntary disclosure to the appropriate law enforcement or regulatory agency.

POLICY

1. Employees, volunteers, physicians, or vendors should report any potential violations of federal, state, or local laws or regulations to their immediate supervisor/manager and to the compliance officer.

2. If misconduct is reported or detected, the organization will determine, via inquiry and investigation, whether credible evidence exists to indicate that a violation of criminal, civil, or administrative law has occurred.

3. If the organization determines that credible evidence of a legal violation exists, it will respond to the offense by developing a corrective action initiative and, if deemed necessary, by disclosing the misconduct to the appropriate third-party law enforcement or regulatory agency.

4. The OIG will be notified in writing, within 30 days of the date of discovery, of any ongoing investigation or legal proceeding conducted or brought by a governmental entity or its agents involving an allegation that the organization has committed a crime or has engaged in fraudulent activities or any other knowing misconduct.

5. The OIG will be notified in writing, within 30 days, if, after reasonable inquiry, the organization discovers credible evidence of misconduct that may violate criminal, civil, or administrative law concerning the organization's practices relating to the federal healthcare programs.

6. Any inquiries and/or investigations will be conducted in an expeditious manner to ensure that all requisite reporting is accomplished in accordance with any legal or regulatory guidelines.

PROCEDURES

1. Anyone with knowledge of a potential violation of law or regulation, particularly a situation that may require return of prior payments, should report that information to his/her immediate supervisor/manager, who, in turn, will report the matter to the compliance officer.

2. The compliance officer will determine what further investigation is required, such as auditing or monitoring of the situation, or additional training of personnel, or the rebilling or refunding of a claim. The compliance officer will also make arrangements for the appropriate actions/procedures.

3. The compliance officer and/or legal counsel will conduct appropriate inquiries and investigations into reports of misconduct that may include violations of civil, criminal, or administrative law (see Compliance Office and Legal Counsel Policy on CD-ROM Template 2-2-9).

4. Legal counsel will supervise and direct compliance investigations into allegations that indicate a violation of law.

5. Corrective action may include voluntary disclosure or reporting of violations of civil, criminal, or administrative law to appropriate third-party law enforcement or regulatory agencies.

6. Legal counsel, in consultation with the compliance officer, will present findings and

recommendations to senior management to ensure that proper corrective action is taken and, if necessary, that the violation is disclosed to an appropriate third party.

7. If after reasonable inquiry and investigation, the compliance officer and/or senior management believe that any misconduct constitutes a violation of the False Claims Act, a report should be made to the appropriate civil and/or criminal law enforcement agency within 30 days.

REFERENCES/CITATIONS

OIG Compliance Program Guidance for Hospitals. Published by the Office of Inspector General in a *Federal Register* notice, dated February 23, 1998, and Supplemental Compliance Guidance January 31, 2005 (see 70 *FR* 4858). Available at the OIG Web site: *http://oig.hhs.gov/authorities/docs/cpghosp.pdf.*

Disclosure of Overpayments and Deficiencies

Part of any appropriate corrective action is the prompt identification and restitution of any overpayment to the affected payer immediately upon discovery, as well as the imposition of proper disciplinary action. Failure to repay overpayments within a reasonable period of time could be interpreted as an intentional attempt to conceal the overpayment from the government, thereby establishing an independent basis for a criminal violation to the organization, as well as any individuals who may have been involved.

For this reason, according to the OIG, compliance programs should emphasize that overpayments obtained from Medicare or other federal healthcare programs will be promptly returned to the payer who made the erroneous payment. An additional template relating to overpayments, Template 26, *Disclosure of overpayments and deficiencies,* is available on the accompanying bonus CD-ROM (Template 2-5-26). The sample policy template follows the suggested course of action offered by the OIG.

Compliance Element 6: Auditing and monitoring

The OIG defines auditing and monitoring as "an ongoing evaluation process [that] is critical to a successful compliance program." They accept the fact that there are many monitoring techniques available, including periodic compliance audits by internal or external auditors who have expertise in federal and state healthcare statutes, regulations, and federal healthcare program requirements.

Monitoring techniques suggested by the OIG include sampling protocols that permit the compliance officer to identify and review compliance risk areas. They also state:

> An effective compliance program should also incorporate periodic (at least annual) reviews of whether the program's compliance elements have been satisfied, e.g., whether there has been appropriate dissemination of the program's standards, training, ongoing education programs and disciplinary actions, among others.

The use of audits and/or other evaluation techniques to monitor compliance and assist in the reduction of identified problem areas is one of the seven essential elements for an effective compliance program.

There are two general types of auditing and monitoring requirements for a compliance program. First, the compliance officer is responsible for ensuring that the elements of the program remain effective. For example, the compliance officer should periodically audit the employee hotline to ensure that employees are aware of its existence and are willing to us it. Also, the compliance officer should review the hotline to ensure that operations are in accordance with established policies and procedures. Second, the compliance officer must ensure that areas of risk are monitored consistently and appropriately.

The OIG believes an ongoing evaluation process is critical to a successful compliance program. An effective program should incorporate thorough monitoring of its implementation and regular reporting to senior or corporate officers. Compliance reports created by this ongoing monitoring, including reports of suspected non-compliance, should be maintained by the compliance officer and shared with senior management and the compliance committee. The OIG recommends that these audits and reviews should include but not be limited to the following:

1. Focus on all programs or divisions, including external relationships with third-party contractors, specifically those with substantive exposure to government enforcement actions

2. Be designed to address compliance with laws governing kickback arrangements, coding, claim development and submission, reimbursement, cost reporting, and marketing

3. Address compliance with specific regulations, rules and policies

4. Include monitoring techniques such as sampling protocols that create a baseline audit of items and services, with provisions to identify and act on significant variations from the baseline

5. Include periodic reviews to determine if the compliance program's elements have been satisfied (e.g,. initial training, ongoing education, disciplinary actions, etc.)

6. Include on-site visits, interviews with key people in management, operations, and coding

7. Use employee surveys designed to solicit impressions of a broad cross-section of staff members

8. Review medical/financial records and other source documents that support claims for reimbursement

9. Engage in trend analyses/longitudinal studies that seek deviations from established patterns

It is not necessarily the compliance officer's responsibility to conduct audits. In fact, this may be outside his or her level of expertise. However, the compliance officer can coordinate with the proper resources (e.g., inside or outside auditors) to accomplish auditing and monitoring responsibilities.

Monitoring the overall compliance program

Monitoring techniques may include sampling protocols that permit the compliance officer to identify and review variations from an established baseline. Significant variations from the baseline should trigger a reasonable inquiry to determine the cause of the deviation.

If the inquiry determines that the deviation occurred for legitimate, explainable reasons, the compliance officer, administrator, or manager may want to limit any corrective action or take no action. However, if it is determined that the deviation was caused by improper procedures or a misunderstanding of rules, including fraud and systemic problems, the organization should take prompt steps to correct the problem.

The OIG notes that as part of the review process, the compliance officer or reviewers should consider techniques such as:

- On-site visits

- Interviews with management and employees in all activities of the organization

- Soliciting impressions of the employees and staff using questionnaires

- Reviewing records that support claims for reimbursement

- Reviewing written materials and documentation relating to business practices

- Conducting trend analyses and studies to identify deviations in practices

The OIG believes reviewers must:

- Be independent of line management

- Have access to existing relevant documents and people

- Report results to the CEO, governing body, and compliance committee

- Specifically identify areas where corrective actions are needed

With these reports, management personnel can take whatever steps they deem necessary to correct past problems and prevent them from recurring. In certain cases, subsequent reviews or studies would be advisable to ensure that the recommended corrective actions have been implemented successfully. The organization should document its efforts to comply with applicable statutes, regulations, and federal healthcare program requirements.

For example, where an organization, in its efforts to comply with a particular statute, regulation, or program requirement, requests advice from a government agency (including a Medicare fiscal intermediary or carrier) charged with administering a federal healthcare program, the organization should document and retain a record of the request and any written or oral response. This step is extremely important if the organization intends to rely on that response to guide it in future decisions, actions, or claim-reimbursement requests or appeals.

Maintaining a log of oral inquiries between the organization and third parties represents an additional basis for establishing documentation on which the organization may rely to demonstrate attempts at compliance. Records should be maintained demonstrating reasonable reliance and due diligence in developing procedures that implement such advice.

The OIG recommends that when a compliance program is established, the compliance officer, with the assistance of department managers, should benchmark the organization from a compliance perspective. This assessment can be undertaken by outside consultants or internal staff members who possess authoritative knowledge of healthcare compliance requirements. This benchmark becomes a baseline for the compliance officer and other managers to ensure that the basic elements of the compliance program are operating effectively.

As part of the review process, the compliance officer should consider techniques such as on-site visits and interviews with personnel involved in management, operations, coding, claim development and submission, patient care, and other related activities. The OIG suggests the employment of question-naires developed to solicit impressions of a broad cross-section of the employees and staff.

Best-practice tip

An effective compliance program should incorporate periodic (at least annual) reviews to de-termine whether the program's compliance elements have been satisfied (e.g., whether there has been appropriate dissemination of the program's standards, training, ongoing educational programs and disciplinary actions, among others). This process will verify actual conformance by all departments with the compliance program. Such reviews could support a determination that appropriate records have been created and maintained to document the implementation of an effective program.

However, when monitoring discloses that deviations were not detected in a timely manner due to program deficiencies, appropriate modifications must be implemented. Such evaluations, when developed with the support of management, can help ensure compliance with the policies and procedures.

Auditing risk areas

One effective tool to promote and ensure compliance is the performance of regular, periodic compli-ance audits by internal or external auditors who have expertise in federal and state healthcare statutes, regulations, and federal healthcare program requirements. The audits should focus on the programs or divisions, including external relationships with third-party contractors, specifically those with substan-tive exposure to government enforcement actions.

At a minimum, these audits should be designed to address the compliance with laws governing:

- Kickback arrangements

- The physician self-referral prohibition

- CPT/HCPCS/ICD-9 coding

- Claim development and submission

- Reimbursement

- Cost reporting

- Marketing

In addition, the audits and reviews should examine the organization's compliance with specific rules and policies that have been the focus of the Medicare fiscal intermediaries or carriers, and law enforcement, as evidenced by OIG Special Fraud Alerts, OIG audits and evaluations, and law enforcement initiatives. The organization should also focus on any areas of concern that have been identified by any entity (i.e., federal, state, or internal) that may apply to the organization.

Monitoring techniques may include sampling protocols that permit the compliance officer to identify and review variations from an established baseline. Significant variations from the baseline should trigger a reasonable inquiry to determine the cause of the deviation. If the inquiry determines that the deviation occurred for legitimate, explainable reasons, the compliance officer, administrator, or manager may want to limit any corrective action or take no action.

If it is determined that the deviation was caused by improper procedures or misunderstanding of rules, including fraud and systemic problems, the organization should take prompt steps to correct the problem. Any overpayments discovered as a result of such deviations should be returned promptly to the affected payer, with appropriate documentation and a thorough explanation for the reason behind the refund.

The OIG understands the variances and complexities within the industry and is sensitive to the differences among large urban medical centers; community organizations; small, rural organizations; specialty hospitals; and other types of hospital organizations and systems. The OIG recognizes that some organizations may not be able to adopt certain elements to the same comprehensive degree that others with more-extensive resources may achieve.

The OIG guidances suggest how an organization can best establish internal controls and monitoring to correct and prevent fraudulent activities. However, by no means should the contents of the OIG guidances be viewed as an exclusive discussion of the advisable elements of a compliance program.

An ongoing auditing and monitoring process should include regular reporting of results to senior or corporate officers. The compliance officer's primary responsibilities should include overseeing and monitoring the implementation of the compliance program. Compliance reports created by this ongoing monitoring, including reports of suspected non-compliance, should be maintained by the compliance officer and shared with the senior management and the compliance committee. The regular auditing and monitoring of the compliance activities must be a key feature in any annual review. Appropriate reports on audit findings should be periodically provided and explained to a parent organization's senior staff and officers.

A sample policy and procedure, Template 27, *Auditing and monitoring high-risk areas,* is included on this book's bonus CD-ROM (Template 2-6-27)

Auditing the compliance program for effectiveness

An ongoing evaluation process is critical to a successful compliance program. The OIG believes that an effective program should incorporate thorough monitoring of its implementation and regular reporting to senior or corporate officers. Compliance reports created by this ongoing monitoring, including reports of suspected non-compliance, should be maintained by the compliance officer and shared with the senior management and the compliance committee.

An effective compliance program should also incorporate periodic (at least annual) reviews of whether the program's compliance elements have been satisfied (e.g., whether there has been appropriate dissemination of the program's standards, training, ongoing educational programs, and disciplinary actions, among others). This process will verify actual conformance by all departments with the compliance program. Such reviews could support a determination that appropriate records have been created and maintained to document the implementation of an effective program.

However, when monitoring discloses that deviations were not detected in a timely manner due to program deficiencies, appropriate modifications must be implemented. Such evaluations, when developed with the support of management, can help ensure compliance with the policies and procedures.

TEMPLATE 28:

AUDITING AND MONITORING THE COMPLIANCE PROGRAM

DEPARTMENT: COMPLIANCE OFFICE	EFFECTIVE DATE:
POLICY NUMBER:	APPROVAL DATE:
POLICY: Auditing and Monitoring of the Compliance Program	APPROVED BY:
POLICY REPLACED:	NUMBER OF PAGES:

BACKGROUND

We have developed and implemented a compliance program in an effort to establish, in part, effective internal controls that promote adherence to applicable federal and state law and to the program requirements of federal, state, and private health plans, as called for by the OIG in its compliance guidance documents. An ongoing evaluation process is critical to a successful compliance program.

One of the compliance officer's primary responsibilities is overseeing and monitoring the implementation of the compliance program. The OIG has noted that periodically revising the program in light of changes in the needs of the organization, and in the law and policies and procedures of government and private payers, is critical to maintaining an effective compliance program.

PURPOSE

To provide guidance on reviewing the effectiveness of the compliance program.

POLICY

1. The executive compliance committee has responsibility for providing oversight of the compliance officer and compliance program.

2. The executive compliance committee will engage an internal or external independent reviewer to review those operations under direction of the compliance officer, such as the handling of hotline information and regular reporting to the compliance committee of the board of

directors on the state of the compliance program and the adequacy of oversight efforts for compliance in the various operations of the organization.

3. The executive compliance committee will annually report the results of the independent reviewer to the compliance committee of the board of directors, along with recommendations to correct any deficiencies noted. These reports will also address the adequacy of resources for sustaining the compliance program operations.

4. The compliance officer is responsible for ensuring that the compliance program is subject to ongoing auditing and monitoring for effectiveness and will report to the executive compliance committee and board of directors annually on all the elements of the compliance program to ensure that they are operating effectively to reduce the likelihood of wrongful acts and non-compliance with applicable regulations. These reports will note all program deficiencies and weaknesses, along with specific recommendations for corrective action.

5. The compliance officer will oversee the use of audits and/or other evaluation techniques to monitor compliance in the various operations, functions and systems of the organization. The results of these reviews will be presented to the executive compliance committee and board of directors at least annually, along with specific recommendations for corrective action measures.

PROCEDURES

1. The executive compliance committee will ensure that an independent auditing and monitoring review of the compliance officer and related operations is executed to determine whether the OIG compliance standards are being met. The findings, citing weaknesses and deficiencies, will be included in a report to the board of directors, along with specific recommendations for corrective action measures for program improvement. These independent reviews will address the following:

   • Has the compliance officer kept the executive compliance committee and board of directors informed on all material facts relating to the compliance program in written reports and briefings that address the progress of implementation? Has the compliance officer assisted in establishing methods to improve the efficiency and quality of services, and has he or she reduced the vulnerability to fraud, abuse, and waste?

   • Has the compliance officer offered appropriate remedial action plans for addressing deficiencies noted in carrying out the duties of the compliance program, including proposed compliance policies modifications, additions and deletions? Has he or she improved internal controls, auditing and monitoring improvements, and specific corrective measures?

- Has the compliance officer adequately developed, coordinated, and participated in compliance educational and training programs that focus on the elements of the compliance program, identifying high-risk areas and seeking to ensure that all appropriate employees and managers are knowledgeable of, and comply with, pertinent federal and state standards?

- Has the compliance officer assisted financial management in coordinating internal compliance review and monitoring activities, including annual or periodic reviews of departments for high-risk areas?

- Has the compliance officer independently investigated and acted on matters related to compliance, with the flexibility to design and coordinate internal investigations of suspected violations of law, regulations, and any resulting corrective action with all departments, providers, sub-providers, agents, and, if appropriate, independent contractors?

- Are there adequate policies and programs to encourage managers and employees to report suspected fraud and other improprieties without fear of retaliation?

- Has management in all departments conducted compliance reviews, with guidance and assistance from the compliance officer, of all high-risk issues within their area of responsibility, with corrective action measures for any deficiencies noted?

- Has the compliance officer verified completion of compliance reviews by management?

- Has the compliance officer verified that corrective action measures arising from compliance reviews have been implemented and tested?

- Has the compliance officer validated corrective measures implemented in the previous year that address any weaknesses identified?

- Has the compliance officer met the responsibility for the proper handling of hotline information consistent with the hotline program's objectives?

- Are all callers to the hotline given the same ground rules, including the right to report anonymously or in confidence without fear of retribution and retaliation?

- Does the compliance officer ensure proper record retention procedures for documents (both electronic and hard copy), and are those records maintained in a secure area, in accordance with records-maintenance policy and best practices?

- Does the compliance officer ensure that the identity of callers and other confidential information appearing on logs and in summary documents is not improperly disclosed?

- Does the compliance officer have a system to log and track all hotline call reports, as well as other reports to the compliance office?

- Has the compliance officer ensured that all call reports have been thoroughly reviewed, appropriate recommendations made, and identified corrective actions completed?

- Do the hotline records show:

  - That the reports are reviewed in a timely manner?

  - Proper referral to appropriate managers with a request and deadline?

  - That all allegations are appropriately handled and investigated?

  - That all issues are resolved in accordance with established procedures, including recommending corrective action and ensuring that such action has been implemented?

- Has the compliance officer ensured that information regarding the hotline in the code of conduct, compliance training materials, hotline posters, corporate newsletters, and other communications channels is accurate and adequate for informing employees and others of the availability of the hotline?

- Do employees view the hotline as a viable communications channel?

- Are logs and summary documents related to hotline information and investigations properly secured to ensure that anonymity and confidentiality of callers are not disclosed by such information?

- Has the compliance officer handled promptly, investigated, and appropriately resolved information derived from the hotline and other sources?

- Did the compliance officer keep the executive compliance committee and board of directors informed on the results of any hotline or other compliance office investigations?

- Has the compliance officer ensured that:

- The facsimile and e-mail systems provide the necessary security in the transmission of reports from the hotline vendor?

- The compliance office space affords the necessary security to deny access to compliance office facsimile machines, computers, records, and other confidential resources when staff members are not present?

- There is proper security over all confidential information resulting from hotline calls?

2. The compliance officer auditing and monitoring will verify that the following questions will be addressed in a report to the executive compliance committee and board of directors:

   • What is the adequacy of compliance office policies and procedures? Are new compliance policies needed? Do existing ones require modification? Should any policies be retired or eliminated?

   • Have the code of conduct and other written compliance policies and procedures that promote commitment to compliance been distributed to all new employees?

   • Do all manager and employee performance plans include adherence to compliance as an element of evaluations?

   • Have department managers met their obligations for ongoing auditing and monitoring of high-risk issues relating to their area (e.g., areas of potential fraud, such as claims development and submission processes, code gaming, and financial relationships with physicians and other healthcare professionals)?

   • Have department managers provided specific recommendations for corrective action measures or program improvement, such as development and proposed additions, deletions, or modifications to compliance office policies and procedures that address noted deficiencies?

   • Are all new employees, business associates, and vendors screened against the OIG's List of Excluded Individuals and Entities (LEIE) and the GSA Debarment List?

   • Have all independent contractors and agents who furnish medical services to the organization been made aware of the requirements of the compliance program?

- Has the compliance officer reported to the executive compliance committee and board of directors on the general status and outcome of operational compliance auditing and monitoring?

REFERENCES/CITATIONS

OIG Compliance Program Guidance for Hospitals. Published by the Office of Inspector General in a *Federal Register* notice, dated February 23, 1998, and Supplemental Compliance Guidance January 31, 2005 (see 70 *FR* 4858). Available at the OIG Web site: *http://oig.hhs.gov/authorities/docs/cpghosp.pdf.*

A sample review guide, Template 29, *Compliance program review guide,* is available on the accompanying bonus CD-ROM (Template 2-6-29).

Hotline auditing and monitoring for effectiveness

Another area for auditing and monitoring involves the hotline operation. By definition, the hotline is an effective communications channel for employees to use to report problems and concerns and is a critical aspect of an effective compliance program.

If a hotline is established to provide this communications channel, the compliance officer should routinely audit and monitor the hotline to ensure that it operates in accordance with established policy. Employees should feel comfortable contacting the hotline and should understand that all calls will be reviewed and taken seriously. This policy is designed to provide the compliance officer with guidance on how and when to conduct formal hotline audits

Over recent years, there has been an ever-increasing move towards having an employee hotline, including the Sentencing Commission Guidelines, OIG compliance guidance documents, Sarbanes-Oxley Act, HIPAA, and Supreme Court decisions on sexual harassment, among others.

The OIG in its various compliance guidance documents stresses not only the importance of compliance communication and hotlines as a critical element of any compliance program but also that such a program should be *effective*. The problem for many is trying to determine what an effective hotline function should look like.

It is important to conduct an independent review or review of the hotline operation periodically to determine:

- Whether the hotline is operating in accordance with the established protocols, policies, and procedures

- The level of documentation and evidence of the operation is adequate to ensure effectiveness

- Whether stated objectives for the hotline operation are being achieved

Scope of reviews

Reviews should focus on whether the hotline is being operated in a manner consistent with the established protocols, policies, and procedures designed for its operation.

Audit steps include:

- An on-site visit to where hotline information is received processed, stored, transmitted, and managed

- Visible examination of the security of the files

- Drawing and examining a sample of files for compliance with existing written policies and procedures

- Examining reports on hotline operation provided to senior managers and executives—including those at the board of director's level—for content and accuracy

Auditing the call log

The hotline should be available through a toll-free number that cannot be traced back to the caller. The hotline call log should be examined to ensure that it includes specific information for each call taken, including:

- Caller identification number

- Identifying initials of the operator taking the call

- Date the call was received

- Whether investigation of the call information is required (yes or no)

- Whether the investigation is completed (yes or no)

- Whether follow-up action is needed (yes or no)

- Whether follow-up has been completed (yes or no)

- Date of resolution

Auditing the hotline manual

Organizations with a hotline should have policies and procedures governing all aspects of the function gathered in a single manual that provides instructions and guidance on the operation of the hotline. The annual review of this hotline manual should verify that the policies:

- Provide adequate guidance to those taking hotline calls

- Are written in a clear and concise manner

- Have been distributed to all those involved in the operation, including those within the organization and, if the answering is contracted out to a vendor, to their people as well

The manual review should ensure that the policies provide guidance on each of the following:

1. Types of routine and investigative compliance services

2. General compliance reviews

3. Conducting investigations

4. Phone procedures for receiving hotline calls

5. General operating protocols

6. Documentation and tracking of calls

7. Recordkeeping and numbering

8. File retention

9. Closure of cases

10. Contact list of key individuals who may need to be alerted to a call situation

The review should also define the major roles and responsibilities of the hotline, such as to:

- Provide clear and concise statements regarding the operation and objectives of the hotline and describe its operation

- Aid the compliance program in detecting violations of the policies/procedures, organization code of conduct, regulations, and laws

- Provide an outlet for employees to call with issues they perceive to be a problem

- Answer all incoming calls during operating hours, but preferably 24 hours/day

- Ensure that all calls are handled according to predetermined policies and procedures

- Ensure thatcallers are shown empathy and given an opportunity to communicate their concerns

- Provide detailed description of protocols for taking calls, including important questions to ask in the course of a hotline call

The audit should take steps to find evidence that the organization encourages employees to report problems. It should also find evidence that the organization is accepting of reported employee concerns or allegations of suspected violation of law, regulation, organization policy, wrongful behavior, and un-ethical conduct within the organization in the event that the existing management and human resources grievance procedures are inappropriate or unresponsive.

The results of an annual review should be reported in concise, clear statements. The attached CD-ROM includes examples (Figure 2-6-1) of how to show an effective annual hotline audit.

HOTLINE AUDITING AND MONITORING

DEPARTMENT: COMPLIANCE OFFICE	EFFECTIVE DATE:
POLICY NUMBER:	APPROVAL DATE:
POLICY: Hotline Auditing and Monitoring Policy	APPROVED BY:
POLICY REPLACED:	

BACKGROUND

One of the primary responsibilities of the compliance office is to ensure that the hotline operates in conformance with its objectives (see Hotline Policy). Periodic audits of the hotline operation will provide the organization assurances that the hotline is operating in conformance with established procedures.

PURPOSE

To ensure that the hotline is operating effectively through a process of periodic auditing and monitoring.

POLICY

1. The compliance officer has primary responsibility for the hotline operations and will therefore arrange for an independent review of the function at least annually to ensure adherence to established policy and procedures.

2. The report of independent review of the hotline function will be given to the executive compliance committee and the board of directors.

3. The compliance officer will take necessary steps to ensure all findings from the independent review are acted upon with appropriate corrective measures.

PROCEDURES

1. The compliance officer will arrange for periodic independent audits and/or reviews of all aspects of the hotline operation.

2. The audit or review will focus on ensuring the following:

- All calls are answered promptly during established hotline hours

- A pre-recorded message explaining the ground rules of the hotline is in place

- Callers are fully debriefed

- Callers are provided a report identification number

- Callers are not traceable (calls cannot be identified on the telephone bill)

- Call information is kept confidential

- Calls cannot be overheard or seen by the general population

- Record-retention policy is followed

- Records are maintained in a secure area

- Followup on call information is handled promptly and appropriately

- Call logs are maintained properly

- Non-retaliation/Non-retribution policy is followed

- Hotline is viewed by employees as a viable communications channel

3. The compliance officer will provide reports on the results of any hotline audits to the executive compliance committee that, in turn, will report to the board of directors.

4. The compliance officer will make recommendations to the executive compliance committee for any necessary changes to the hotline operation.

REFERENCES/CITATIONS

OIG Compliance Program Guidance for Hospitals. Published by the Office of Inspector General in a *Federal Register* notice, dated February 23, 1998, and Supplemental Compliance Guidance January 31, 2005 (see 70 *FR* 4858). Available at the OIG Web site: *http://oig.hhs.gov/authorities/docs/cpghosp.pdf.*

Auditing and monitoring: Response, followup, and resolution

According to the OIG, one of the seven essential elements for an effective compliance program is the investigation and remediation of identified systemic problems. The compliance officer bears the responsibility for auditing and monitoring and for ensuring that identified risks or problems are corrected or brought into compliance. This comprehensive policy lays out guidelines for remediation of risk areas identified though compliance audits, and it provides a continuing plan for future monitoring and reporting.

TEMPLATE 31:

AUDIT RESOLUTION

DEPARTMENT: COMPLIANCE OFFICE	EFFECTIVE DATE:
POLICY NUMBER:	APPROVAL DATE:
POLICY: AUDIT RESOLUTION	APPROVED BY:
POLICY REPLACED:	NUMBER OF PAGES:

BACKGROUND

Reviews and findings may arise from ongoing auditing and monitoring, independent audits, responses to hotline complaints, etc. The audit review and follow-up process is an integral part of good management, and it is a shared responsibility of management officials, auditors, and reviewers. The issue remains the same—proper resolution of any findings.

This policy specifies the role of the designated officials with regard to followup and strengthens the procedures for ensuring that appropriate action is taken in response to reviews or audit findings, including corrective action on recommendations contained in audit/review reports. This policy emphasizes the importance of monitoring the implementation of resolved audit recommendations to ensure that promised corrective actions are actually taken.

PURPOSE

To establish procedures for responding to findings in reports issued by the internal or external auditors, consultants, or reviews by internal staff.

POLICY

1. Corrective action taken by management on resolved findings and recommendations is essential to improving the effectiveness and efficiency of the organization's operations, as well as ensuring that identified problems and weaknesses do not recur.

2. It is expected that auditors/reviewers will provide responsible managers a comprehensive report and a briefing on their findings and recommendations.

3. The compliance officer will provide oversight of audit resolution, including the receipt of reports from audits or reviews, and evidence of being informed of scheduled meetings wherein management is briefed on the results of such audits/reviews.

4. The compliance officer will maintain a tracking system for compliance-related findings arising from audits or reviews, and he/she is responsible for ensuring that they are tracked until corrective action and follow-up verification are completed.

5. The resolution process will include all actions required to fully correct all issues. Depending on the nature of the problems involved, each resolution will include timely correction of management, system and program compliance issues/deficiencies, monitoring to ensure that the corrective actions on significant deficiencies have been adequately implemented to resolve the problem and ensure that it does not recur, and verification that the corrective actions are operating effectively.

PROCEDURES

1. Resolution is normally deemed to occur when corrective action has been instituted and independently verified.

2. Resolution should take place within 60 days of significant findings being reported. However, if findings indicate the existence of legal or regulatory issues, managers must notify the compliance officer and resolve findings within 30 days.

3. Management officials will maintain audit/review resolution files or other appropriate records to fully document and justify all actions taken to resolve the findings within their area of responsibility. The documentation must specify the target dates for implementation of corrective actions on deficiencies or weaknesses, identify the procedures followed, and document the results of follow-up reviews.

4. Documentation of resolution must be in sufficient detail to satisfy an independent reviewer that the findings have been fully, effectively, and appropriately resolved.

5. Managers of units subjected to review are responsible for monitoring the implementation of actions to correct deficiencies until the deficiencies have been corrected.

- The review should be initiated as soon as possible after corrective actions are implemented.

- The manager may conduct the follow-up review personally or may request that it be conducted by another party (e.g., internal auditor, external auditor, consultant, or personnel from another unit). In any case, he or she must ensure that the party selected possesses the capability of performing the review.

- When significant compliance issues are involved, the compliance officer will independently conduct a follow-up review to ensure that corrective actions taken are effective in preventing recurrence of the problem.

- The manager is ultimately responsible for ensuring that reviews are conducted and for determining whether the deficiencies were adequately corrected.

- Issues and significant deficiencies will not be considered resolved until the manager determines that the actions were in fact taken, and resulted in correction of the deficiencies.

6. At a minimum, managers will submit monthly reports to the compliance officer and their senior management on the actions taken to resolve significant findings and the status of each open finding.

7. The compliance officer will review the reports and follow up with managers as needed.

8. The compliance officer will make regular reports to the compliance committee and the board on the status of all actions.

REFERENCES/CITATIONS

OIG Compliance Program Guidance for Hospitals. Published by the Office of Inspector General in a *Federal Register* notice, dated February 23, 1998, and Supplemental Compliance Guidance January 31, 2005 (see 70 *FR* 4858). Available at the OIG Web site: *http://oig.hhs.gov/authorities/docs/cpghosp.pdf.*

Compliance Element 7: Sanction screening

The OIG suggests that organizations use screening mechanisms to preclude employing or engaging in business relationships with individuals and entities previously convicted of criminal violations or formerly the subject of sanctioning, debarment, exclusion, or other adverse action that could affect their compliance with applicable laws and regulations. Organizations are responsible for those whom they hire, to whom they give discretionary authority, and with whom they do business.

Employing or doing business with sanctioned individuals or entities may result in liability for an organization. Any claim emanating from a sanctioned individual or entity may be viewed as a false claim. A Medicare Part A cost report that includes sanctioned individuals also may be viewed as false. Therefore, organizations should conduct appropriate screening to ensure that they do not employ or do business with individuals or entities that are convicted of criminal violations or have been the subject of sanctioning, debarment, exclusion, or other adverse action that could have an impact on their compliance with applicable laws and regulations.

Employee applications should include questions pertaining to any pending charge or conviction for violation of criminal law and/or any sanction or disciplinary actions by any duly authorized regulatory or enforcement agency of government. It should be the responsibility of any hiring authority to verify the accuracy and honesty of the responses provided by applicants.

The compliance officer should coordinate with human resource management to ensure that the OIG Cumulative Sanction Report has been checked with respect to all employees, medical staff, and independent contractors. An organization should enact policies and procedures that ensure that it will not employ or engage in business with anyone who is currently under sanction or exclusion by any duly authorized enforcement agency or licensing and disciplining authority.

This should be in furtherance of the organization's goal of ensuring that all employees are properly credentialed, licensed, and without a history of misconduct or performance problems. As such, potentially, this type of history may evidence their ability to perform their fiduciary duties and responsibilities in accordance with all applicable requirements including the conditions of participation in Medicare and Medicaid and other government programs.

Prior to hiring new employees who will have discretionary authority to make decisions that may involve compliance with the law or compliance oversight, organizations should conduct a reasonable and prudent background investigation, including a reference check. The application should specifically require the applicant to disclose any criminal conviction as defined by 42 U.S.C. § 1320a-7(i) or any exclusion action.

Pursuant to the compliance program, policies should prohibit the employment of individuals who have been recently convicted of a criminal offense related to healthcare or who are listed as debarred, excluded, or otherwise ineligible for participation in federal healthcare programs (as defined in 42 U.S.C. § 1320a-7b(f)).

In addition, pending the resolution of any criminal charges or proposed debarment or exclusion, the OIG recommends that such individuals be removed from direct responsibility for, or involvement in, any federal healthcare program. With regard to current employees or independent contractors, if resolution of the matter results in conviction, debarment, or exclusion, the organization should terminate its employment or other contract arrangement with the individual or contractor.

The federal government maintains two lists of individuals and entities that have been sanctioned by the government:

- The List of Excluded Individuals and Entities (LEIE) can be found on the Internet at *www.oig. hhs.gov*. It is updated on a regular basis to reflect the status of healthcare providers who have been excluded from participation in the Medicare and Medicaid programs.

- The General Services Administration maintains a monthly listing of debarred contractors on the Internet at *www.arnet.gov/epls*.

The OIG expects healthcare organizations to screen their employees and business partners against these databases to ensure that none is under exclusion by the federal government. In addition, hospitals are expected to check physicians against the National Practitioner Data Bank.

Organizations should verify the credentials of medical professionals or entities it employs, or with whom a business relationship has been established, with appropriate licensing and disciplining authorities. This should include any adverse actions taken against the individual that might impair his or her performance of duties or fiduciary responsibilities.

The verification process should include checking against the current LEIE and the GSA Debarment List for sanctioned or excluded individuals or entities. It should include physicians and other licensed medical practitioners, as well as entities that provide health-related goods or services. The organization also should screen for adverse governmental actions and sanctioning all its vendors, entities with which it enters into joint ventures, or affiliates providing ancillary medically related services.

TEMPLATE 32:

SANCTION SCREENING

DEPARTMENT: Compliance Office	EFFECTIVE DATE:
POLICY NUMBER:	APPROVAL DATE:
POLICY: Sanction Screening	APPROVED BY:
POLICY REPLACED:	

BACKGROUND

We recognize that we are responsible for those whom we hire, those to whom we give discretionary authority, and those with whom we do business. This policy has been developed to ensure that all employees are properly credentialed, licensed, and without a history of misconduct or performance problems.

We recognize that, potentially, this type of history may affect an employee's ability to perform his or her fiduciary duties and responsibilities in accordance with all applicable legal, regulatory, and performance requirements. The OIG in its compliance guidance calls for healthcare organizations to develop policies addressing the non-employment or retention of sanctioned individuals.

The OIG strongly advises companies to utilize screening mechanisms to preclude employing or engaging in business relationships with individuals and entities that have been convicted of criminal violations or have been the subject of sanctioning, debarment, exclusion, or other adverse action that could have an impact on their compliance with applicable laws and regulations.

PURPOSE

To ensure that all employees and others with whom we do business are properly credentialed, licensed, and without a history of misconduct or performance problems.

POLICY

1. We will not employ or engage in business with anyone who is currently under sanction or exclusion by any duly authorized enforcement agency or by any licensing and disciplining authority.

2. We will take all reasonable steps to verify that the information provided is accurate.

3. The credentials of medical professionals or entities employed by us or with whom we establish a business relationship will be checked against the current List of Excluded Individuals and Entities (LEIE) and the General Services Administration Debarment List.

4. Human resource management is responsible for carrying out this policy as it relates to hiring of employees.

5. Credentialing committees are responsible for carrying out this policy in granting staff privileges to medical personnel who are not employees.

6. Procurement is responsible for carrying out this policy as it relates to vendors and contractors.

7. The compliance officer is responsible for monitoring this policy for compliance and reporting results annually to the executive compliance committee and the audit and compliance committee of the board of directors, along with any recommendations for remedial actions or improvements to the program.

PROCEDURES

1. The employment application for all new employees with discretionary authority relating to legal compliance (e.g., healthcare providers, billing managers, or supervisors) will include an attestation by the candidate relating to whether he or she has ever been convicted of a crime or sanctioned by a duly authorized regulatory or enforcement agency of government.

2. The following language will appear on all applications:

   - "Have you ever been convicted of any criminal violation of law, or are you now under pending investigation or charges of violation of criminal law? If yes, explain."

   - "Have you been the subject of any adverse action(s) by any duly authorized sanctioning or disciplinary agency for either conduct-based or performance-based actions? If yes, explain."

3. All vendors, joint-venture parties, or affiliates providing ancillary medically related services will be screened for adverse governmental actions and sanctioning.

4. The compliance officer will conduct an annual review of the employment applications and business entities with which we enter into a business relationship to verify that this policy is enforced, and he/she will provide a report of this to the executive compliance committee and the audit and compliance committee of the board of directors, along with any recommendations for improving the process.

REFERENCES/CITATIONS

OIG Compliance Program Guidance for Hospitals. Published by the Office of Inspector General in a *Federal Register* notice, dated February 23, 1998, and Supplemental Compliance Guidance January 31, 2005 (see 70 *FR* 4858). Available at the OIG Web site: *http://oig.hhs.gov/authorities/docs/cpghosp.pdf*.

Credentialing requirements

The OIG expects that healthcare organizations will screen employees and business partners who are credentialed healthcare providers to ensure that they are in current standing with their respective licensing agencies. It is also the responsibility of the organization to verify the credentials of anyone employed or engaged by the organization to deliver healthcare services.

Some people claim to be physicians when they are not, and some physicians lie about their background. The employment of or engagement in business with sanctioned individuals or entities may result in liability for an organization. Any claim emanating from a sanctioned individual or entity might be viewed as a false claim. A Medicare Part A cost report that includes sanctioned individuals might be viewed as false. Therefore, the compliance officer has responsibility for sanction screening, which should be outlined in a compliance policy.

The Joint Commission (formerly The Joint Commission on Accreditation of Healthcare Organizations, or JCAHO) requires every facility it accredits to credential its licensed independent practitioners (LIP). LIPs are defined as those who provide patient care and services without medical direction or supervision. The Joint Commission, CMS, and OIG call for healthcare organizations to credential their practitioners.

The Joint Commission is four core requirements are:

- Current licensure

- Relevant education, training, or experience

- Current competence

- Ability to perform requested privileges

State laws vary as to what practices cover licensed independent practitioners. Normally they include those with limited licenses, allied health practitioners, or physician assistants.

- Health providers must check their credentials to verify training and experience.

- Accrediting bodies require primary source verification of credentials with the state licensing authority to verify information and to avoid forgeries.

- Organizations may use credentialing verification organizations (CVO) to do these checks.

- It is important to maintain on file documentation proving the verifications were made, showing evidence of a primary-source check.

Joint Commission surveyors want to see a report on the verifications the CVO or credentialing office has completed.

Use the accompanying policy, Template 33, *Credentialing policy,* located on this book's bonus CD-ROM (Template 2-7-33), to craft an appropriate policy document.

Chapter 3 | Monitoring, communicating, and responding to government agencies

Centers for Medicare & Medicaid Services communiqués

The Office of Inspector General (OIG) says it should be a matter of policy to conduct audits and reviews of specific rules and polices of attention of the Medicare fiscal intermediaries or carriers. The OIG recommends that the compliance committee assist in analyzing the organization's industry environment, the legal requirements with which it must comply, and specific risk areas in the organization. The changing regulatory environment necessitates that the compliance committee and chief compliance officer keep current on those changes. For example, it is extremely important that healthcare organizations follow changing guidance for the parent agency for Medicare and Medicaid.

The Centers for Medicare & Medicaid Services (CMS) periodically issue communiqués, such as Medicare Bulletins, Medicaid Alerts, and memoranda issued by the fiscal intermediary that offer alerts and advice regarding changes in policy. They also provide clarification for existing regulations or policies. Many organizations believe that establishing policies and procedures to ensure that they keep current on these changes is a necessary part of their compliance program. The related policy, Template 34, *Communiqués from the Centers for Medicare & Medicaid services (CMS) policy,* located on the bonus CD-ROM (Template 3-34), outlines how this can be done.

OIG special fraud alerts

The OIG says there are many monitoring techniques that can be followed, including audits and reviews for compliance. Specific attention should be paid to rules and polices that have been the focus of particular attention on the part of the OIG through their Special Fraud Alerts, audits, and evaluations, as well as enforcement initiatives. The OIG periodically issues these, setting forth activities believed to raise legal and enforcement issues.

Over the years, the OIG has used fraud alerts as a vehicle to identify fraudulent and abusive practices within the healthcare industry. The majority of these fraud alerts are disseminated internally to the OIG's Office of Investigations and other agencies within the Department of Health and Human Services (HHS). The OIG has also developed and issued Special Fraud Alerts intended for extensive distribution directly to the healthcare provider community.

Since 1988, the OIG has issued a number of "Special Fraud Alerts" addressing specific trends of healthcare fraud and certain practices of an industry-wide character. Specifically, the OIG Special Fraud Alerts have served to provide general guidance to the healthcare industry on violations of federal law (including various aspects of the Anti-Kickback Statute), as well as to provide additional insight to the Medicare carrier fraud units in identifying healthcare fraud schemes.

In developing these Special Fraud Alerts, the OIG relies on a number of sources, such as studies or management and program evaluations conducted by the OIG's Office of Evaluation and Inspections. In addition, the OIG may consult with experts in the subject field, including those within the OIG or other agencies.

For the most part, the OIG Special Fraud Alerts have been reserved for national trends in healthcare fraud and have addressed potential violations of the Medicare and state healthcare programs' Anti-Kickback Statute.

The OIG stresses that compliance programs should require that the legal staff, the chief compliance officer, or other appropriate personnel carefully consider any and all Special Fraud Alerts issued by the OIG that relate to the organization's areas of operation. Many of these Special Fraud Alerts are published in the *Federal Register*. The OIG's stated goal and intent is to publicize its concern about possible widespread and abusive healthcare industry practices, and it is seeking wider dissemination of this information to the general public.

A sample policy, Template 35, *OIG Fraud Alerts policy,* is located on the accompanying CD-ROM (Template 3-35). An additional policy also located on the CD-ROM (Template 3-36), Template 36, *Seeking government regulatory guidance policy,* is designed to formulate appropriate channels for compliance inquiries.

Responding to visits by government officials

The federal government conducts numerous investigations and audits of healthcare organizations each year. Most compliance officers and healthcare attorneys do not have an investigative or government-audit background, and they do not understand the government's use of techniques such as unannounced visits to conduct interviews and/or request documents, the service of subpoenas, or the execution of search warrants. Therefore, most healthcare organizations are not prepared to respond appropriately to these events. It is important to develop policies and procedures to cover the following situations:

1. What to do if government officials (e.g., regulators, agents, investigators, auditors, inspectors) make requests for records, interviews, or other "evidence."

2. What to do in response to the following formalized government methods of compelling evidence production:

    • A letter requesting certain records or information

    • A request for a consensual search

    • Service of an Administrative Subpoena for records

    • Service of a Federal Grand Jury Subpoena (two types):

    • Court Order Search Warrants

        – Duces tacum (records to be returned to federal grand jury by specified date)

        – In Personem (compelling appearance of individuals for testimony)

3. Would the presence of regulators at the hospital be considered a critical event?

4. Are you certain that the CEO would be immediately notified in this kind of situation?

5. How do employees know how to react to events?

6. How would you define critical events?

7. How can events be classified to ensure appropriate notification?

8. In the absence of the CEO, how is there a guarantee that procedures will be followed?

9. What critical events already have developed response plans?

10. Discuss how critical events are similar, with similar response needs.

11. How can you test effectiveness of your existing crisis or critical response?

12. Are there elements of the various plans that are common to one another?

13. Are there areas where you believe response plans are needed?

It is increasingly likely that a healthcare provider will come into direct contact with a government regulatory or enforcement agency. It is a good idea to have a response plan for management and staff, or for each type of encounter that might come about. It is logical that this responsibility would fall under the duties of the compliance officers. Needless to say, the OIG compliance guidance does not address this problem because OIG does not see it as a problem.

This part of the book is designed to assist compliance officers in designing appropriate response strategies for a variety of encounters with government agencies. There are any number of events that can lead to a visit by government investigators for conducting interviews, serving subpoenas, arrest warrants, or search warrants. Any of these may arise from the following:

- A routine government audit

- An investigation arising from a computer program or screen design to identify wrongful behavior

- A qui tam action arising from a "whistleblower" or disgruntled employee

- Undercover operation or "sting" operation

- A competitor complaining about unfair business practices

One of the worst things you can do is try to control what employees say and don't say. The government would see that as an obstruction. It is appropriate to tell employees that:

- They are under no obligation to talk to investigators

- The company's attorney can assist them but can't represent them, as that would be a conflict of interest because the attorney represents the company

- They can retain their own attorney

- The company asks that they tell the company's attorney if they are visited by government agents with a subpoena or search warrant

Any of several agencies can come knocking during an investigation—the Federal Bureau of Investigation, (FBI) OIG, Internal Revenue Service, or state agencies. It's important to keep a cool head and to ask for a business card and the name of the agent in charge so you can tell your attorney.

What management should do

A manager should be assigned to show the agents where the information they're authorized to collect is located—but not to answer any questions. The last thing you want is investigators walking around looking for whatever they want. Make sure that they get only what they're supposed to.

Other things to remember:

- Ask for a copy of the warrant and fax it to your attorney.

- Keep a list of what was inspected or copied. That helps your lawyer figure out what the investigation is about.

- Ask for copies of seized documents. Make the argument that these are documents you need to keep your business going.

- Carefully review the warrant—agents can seize only what's listed.

- Point out to the agent if search areas are not listed on the warrant.

- Send all employees—except response coordinator or team—home.

- Do not interfere with investigators. It's a sure way to get arrested.

- Keep documents created under the attorney-client privilege in a separate location. These should be clearly identified and kept separate from other documents the agents are given.

The aftermath

Once the investigators leave, you still have more work to do:

- Ask investigators for a debriefing to try to find out more about the investigation and what they're looking for.

- Consider hiring a public relations firm if media learn of the search.

- Tell employees what's happening, rather than leaving it to the rumor mill.

- Conduct a thorough internal investigation.

- Consider hiring outside consultants.

- If a whistleblower triggered the investigation, the company attorney should contact the whistleblower's attorney and arrange for him or her to stay home at full salary so he or she can't gather documents at work that could be used against the organization. Do **not** fire the whistleblower.

Use the policy included on the CD-ROM (Template 3-37) Template 37, *Responding to visits by government officials policy.*

Responding to subpoenas (DOJ)

The Department of Justice and the OIG routinely use subpoenas to compel the production of documents, records, and other evidence. This tool may also be used in criminal investigations to compel testimony before the Federal Grand Jury (FGJ).

Subpoenas can also be used to compel testimony from potential witnesses. The target of a subpoena must comply with the demand. Failure to produce requested information might result in significant penalties.

Both administrative subpoenas and FGJ subpoenas are enforceable by the U.S. District Courts. Any failure to comply with subpoena demands can result in significant penalties and sanctions up to and including criminal prosecution for contempt of court or possibly obstruction of justice. Additionally, failing to fulfill an administrative subpoena may result in exclusion from government healthcare programs. It is therefore critical that managers and staff understand the process of complying with a subpoena during a government investigation or review.

Subpoenas are being used more frequently in healthcare due to a rise in the number of civil, criminal, and administrative actions against providers of healthcare services and products. The growth in their use is a result of the expanded involvement of regulatory and law enforcement agencies in healthcare investigations.

During healthcare investigations, the government will review records, documents, and accounts to evaluate business practices. It is increasingly common for the government to compel the provision of these company records by issuing subpoenas.

Subpoenas are also used to compel testimony from potential witnesses. The target of a subpoena must comply with the demand. Failure to produce requested information might result in significant penalties.

Therefore, it is important to understand how a subpoena works, how to comply with its demands, and how to protect legal rights. Subpoenas are a less-invasive form of information procurement than search warrants.

Although the level of disruption may be less severe, the implications of failing to comply can be significant. Management and staff should understand the procedures of complying with a subpoena and be advised to assist in the production of demanded information.

Subpoenas are a powerful tool for the government because they may be issued on mere tips or speculation in an effort to gather useful evidence. Healthcare investigations frequently require first-hand accounts, or documentary evidence of fraud or abuse, to support a case. This may require testimony, paper or electronic files, records, reports, accounts, and other data.

There are different types of subpoenas for different uses, including:

- FGJ Subpoenas called "ad testificandum" (compelling testimony before the FGJ)

- FGJ Subpoenas called "duces tecum" (compelling production of records and documents before the FGJ)

- Civil Investigative Demand by the DOJ for evidence and records

- Administrative Subpoena "duces tecum" issued by the OIG (compelling production of records before that office)

FGJ subpoenas are issued in connection with criminal investigations before that body. They are less frequently observed in healthcare investigations. Similarly, Civil Investigative Demands, which are authorized by the DOJ (normally through their U.S. Attorney Offices), are demands for records in connection with civil fraud investigations.

The authority to issue Administrative Subpoenas has been conferred upon the OIG for the Department of Health and Human Services and is commonly used by the OIG in gathering documentary evidence.

They are normally confined to civil and administrative fraud investigations and do not involve compelling testimony. Both administrative subpoenas and FGJ subpoenas are enforceable by the U.S. District Courts.

There are serious personal risks of adverse action against those who fail to obey this order, and it is therefore critical that managers and staff understand the process of complying with a subpoena during a government investigation or review.

Subpoenas are governed by the Fourth Amendment protection against unreasonable or oppressive searches and seizures. Overly broad, irrelevant, or unreasonable requests may be challenged. If the subpoena appears unreasonable or unduly burdensome, it may be legally challenged and an attorney may move to have the subpoena quashed. However, the recipient remains obligated to comply with the subpoena's demands until the issuing court or administrative authority withdraws, changes, or amends the specifications of the subpoena.

It is important that the organization know how to respond to a demand for the production of records, files, and accounts. Someone in the organization should be designated to act as the "custodian of records" and as the contact person in the event of a government investigation or review. This individual should be responsible for collecting the records included in the subpoena. This person should be knowledgeable about the recordkeeping system, policies, and procedures of the office. All production of records for the government should be coordinated with legal counsel.

Upon the receipt of a subpoena, competent legal counsel should immediately be notified and provided a copy of the subpoena along with other pertinent information, such as its mode of delivery. Legal counsel should determine when the subpoena was received, by whom, when the document production and/or appearance to testify is required, and what efforts will be necessary to comply with the subpoena.

It is important to make an initial assessment as to whether the subpoena is specific enough to identify the proper documents, records, or individual for testimony. It is also important to determine whether the time frame for delivery of requested information is reasonable. Legal counsel should also determine whether any of the material sought is protected by privilege (e.g., attorney-client privilege).

Once a subpoena has been served, it is essential that the entire matter be discussed with legal counsel, including possible courses of action. It is also important to inform all members of the staff that no documents should be destroyed or altered during the investigation. Any such action could result in contempt of court or otherwise result in criminal prosecution or additional sanctions.

It is also advisable to conduct an internal inquiry or audit of any issues that may be inferred from the records or information submitted so as to understand the scope of the potential problem with the government. The focus of this effort will help identify potential risks and liabilities and help the organization develop an action plan to respond to possible eventualities. It is inadvisable to try to engage the agents serving subpoenas in conversation, as this may be taken out of context and further complicate matters.

It is critical that production of requested information be made within the established time frame. If this is not feasible, then legal counsel should contact the government to arrange for a delay. It is important to make clear and accurate copies of the original records to be produced.

Provide a complete set of subpoenaed documents to legal counsel and retain a set for daily operation. It is important to note that the government expects the original copies, unless otherwise directed. It is also important to ensure that legal counsel reviews all documents before their release to the government.

Subpoenas avoid the invasive qualities of a search warrant by allowing the recipient to control the production of the requested documents within an allotted time frame. Furthermore, a subpoena provides an opportunity to challenge its demands, such as the scope of records or time allotted to produce materials. This is in contrast to a search warrant, where agents of the government conducting the search seize information on the spot.

TEMPLATE 38:

RESPONDING TO SUBPOENA POLICY

DEPARTMENT: COMPLIANCE OFFICE	EFFECTIVE DATE:
POLICY NUMBER:	APPROVAL DATE:
POLICY: Responding to Subpoena Policy	APPROVED BY:

BACKGROUND

A subpoena is an official demand for testimony or the disclosure of documents or other information (sometimes called "subpoena duces tecum"). Subpoenas are increasingly being used by government agencies in gathering evidence in investigations. The subpoena permits the release of documents that otherwise may not be releasable.

There are two types of subpoenas issued: those by the Federal Grand Jury (FGJ) as part of a criminal investigation and administrative subpoenas issued by law enforcement or administrative agencies in furtherance of either a criminal or a civil investigation. The OIG is one of those agencies that can issue administrative subpoenas.

All subpoenas, regardless of whether they are issued by the FGJ or administrative agency, are enforceable in the U.S. District Court. This is a complicated area that necessitates having procedures for responding to such subpoenas to prevent disruptions to patient services, to ensure that legal counsel coordinates the response, and to guide staff members in their efforts to assist the officers in carrying out the subpoena. Every subpoena requires a careful legal review prior to response. In view of this and the serious legal implications of the receipt of a subpoena, it is necessary to have standing policies and procedures to ensure that legal counsel reviews any subpoena immediately and coordinates the organization's response.

PURPOSE

To provide written guidance on how to respond to a subpoena issued by a duly authorized government agency.

POLICY

1. We are committed to full compliance with any lawful subpoena, and therefore it is our policy that all employees remain courteous and professional when dealing with investigators or agents delivering a subpoena.

2. No one is to impede in any way efforts to deliver a subpoena.

3. If a government agent serves a subpoena, he or she is acting as an agent of a grand jury or conducting an investigation in which an administrative subpoena has been issued, and any interference could be construed as obstruction of justice.

4. Employees will remain courteous and professional when dealing with investigators or agents delivering a subpoena.

5. It is not necessary to volunteer information or to try to instruct investigators on how to do their job.

PROCEDURE

1. When a grand jury subpoena or an administrative subpoena is received, employees should direct the issuer to any individual named in the subpoena or to the person occupying a named position (e.g., Custodian of Records). No other information or discussion should be offered to the agent/investigator. No one should submit to any form of questioning or interviewing at the time of subpoena service.

2. The person accepting the service of the subpoena from the investigators should note all information provided by the investigators (e.g., the name, title, and telephone number of the serving agent/investigator; information provided by the agent/investigator at the time of subpoena service, etc.). Once the agent/investigator has served the subpoena, no other action should be taken until direction is provided from legal counsel.

3. Whoever accepts service of a subpoena should identify the individual at the facility who is most qualified and available to assist legal counsel in responding to the subpoena.

4. The subpoena then must be delivered immediately to the senior manager present in the facility. The manager must be provided with any information obtained during the service of the subpoena.

5. The manager will immediately notify legal counsel of the receipt of the subpoena and any information obtained from investigators, and a facsimile copy will be forwarded immediately.

6. No action should be taken to respond to the subpoena until directions are received from counsel. It is imperative that contact with counsel be immediate if the subpoena is a "forthwith" subpoena commanding an immediate appearance or delivery of documents and records to a federal grand jury.

The compliance office also should be notified and provided with the same information.

Responding to a search warrant

1. Criminal enforcement agencies increasingly have been using search warrants in addition to administrative and FGJ subpoenas in "white-collar" healthcare fraud and abuse investigations. The movement away from use of subpoenas to this more intrusive tool results from their concern that key documents and computerized records might be compromised by written demands for them. A search warrant permits the government to come in and seize records and other evidence forthwith.

2. In view of the serious legal implications of such an event, it is advisable for any compliance officer to have a contingency plan to arrange for immediate notification of designated legal counsel. If relying on outside counsel, it is unlikely they will be present or reach the locale in time to be present during the search and seizure.

3. It is therefore advisable to establish a response plan to such an event, including a set of written internal procedures to assist in dealing with this kind of situation. This should be done in consultation with legal counsel. They will have more specific guidance regarding privileged documents and files.

The following offers some general rules of thumb for consideration.

1. First and foremost, avoid overtly reacting negatively to the agents serving the subpoena.

2. At all times, remain courteous and professional.

3. Try not to impede the agents in any way in executing their orders from the court.

4. Respond to their requests, but do not tell them how to do their business or volunteer information or help them.

5. Remember that the agents may enter into and look at virtually anything in the defined location, including any room, locked cabinets, file, desk drawers, etc. This includes forcing entry to any individual workspace.

6. If government agents arrive with a search warrant, bear in mind that they are acting as agents

of the court. Any interference could well be viewed as obstruction of justice, an actionable offense.

The following are some suggestions for consideration in developing a response plan:

- Identify an outside counsel experienced in health law and federal enforcement who would be on call as needed. Have his or her name and contact information on file.

- Designate someone as the leader of the management response team at each company location. This person should receive the search warrant (or subpoenas) and, in consultation with legal counsel, will interact with the government agents.

- Others should be designated to assist the company in monitoring any search, using a minimum number of people to reduce the level of confusion (the team should include those employees who understand the company's electronic storage and communications systems). As part of their duties, these staff members should reassure employees who could be distressed by the process. Those staff members who are distressed should be removed from the environment as soon as possible.

- Train reception staff members to respond appropriately to government agents when they arrive unannounced. Training should include:

  - To what office or room they should direct the agents.

  - Who to notify to meet them (designated leader as noted above).

  - Possibly also a list of people who should be alerted. Do not leave the agents alone to cool their heels, as they have the legal right to proceed without permission.

A predetermined call list should be in place so that the names on the list can automatically be alerted concerning the search.

Staff members not designated as part of the response team should be removed from the scene and encouraged not to interact with the agents. There is no obligation to give an interview during a search, but it is inadvisable to appear to instruct employees not to talk to agents. The best policy is to just let government agents do their job. Any questions from the agents should be directed to the designated lead person.

The lead person should:

- Meet the agents quickly and inquire politely as to how they may be assisted

- Take note of what agencies are represented and their names (they will identify themselves)

- Make no attempt to copy their credentials (they will rightly object)

- Ask to review the warrant and request a copy

- Work out an agreement to the degree possible of the areas of search as described in the warrant and maintaining reproduced copies of the records seized

- Send a copy of the warrant to legal counsel by the most expeditious means

Additional considerations for lead person:

- The warrant should be carefully examined by the designated lead person (with legal counsel, if present) to determine what specific premises it covers and what specific documents/evidence they seek. Any overt flaw in the warrant should be pointed out to the agents. Politely object to any searches outside the scope of the warrant. Do not interfere should they go ahead and search in the objected area. Note the fact for legal counsel, and any results of the search may later be suppressed.

- It is always advisable to request time before the search to consult with counsel to determine appropriate course of conduct prior to initiation of search. It is likely that the request will not be honored.

- If designated privileged files and documents are on the premises, the government agents in charge of the search need to be notified. If the government agents seize any of these privileged records, make sure the lead employee notes that he or she advised the government agent of that fact.

- The designated team leader should be responsible for maintaining a record of what happens, including number/identity of agents, areas searched, times of search, records/materials taken, etc. This is particularly important if patient records are taken, but they are not exempt from any search.

TEMPLATE 39:	

SEARCH WARRANT POLICY

DEPARTMENT: COMPLIANCE OFFICE	EFFECTIVE DATE:
POLICY NUMBER:	APPROVAL DATE:
POLICY: Search Warrant Policy	APPROVED BY:

BACKGROUND

Federal and state law enforcement agencies are increasingly using search warrants in conjunction with healthcare fraud investigations. A search warrant permits agents to seize documents and other types of information immediately.

The movement away from use of subpoenas to this more intrusive tool results from the government's concern that key documents and computerized records might be compromised by written demands for them. A search warrant permits the government to come in and seize records and other evidence forthwith.

In view of the serious legal implications of such an event, it is necessary to have standing policy and procedures to arrange for immediate notification of designated legal counsel. It is unlikely that he or she will be present or reach the locale in time to be present during the search and seizures. It is therefore important to establish a response plan to such an event, including a set of written internal procedures to assist in dealing with this kind of situation.

The execution of a search warrant can be seriously disruptive and frightening for many employees. Furthermore, if not handled properly, an organization subject to a search warrant may compound its problems.

PURPOSE

The purpose of this policy is to provide written guidance on how to respond appropriately to an official search warrant.

POLICY

1. It is our policy that at all times employees will remain courteous and professional in dealing with agents and officers of the court who are serving search warrant orders. No one is permitted to impede the agents or interfere in any way with the lawful execution of a search warrant.

2. Each separate geographic unit in the organization will establish one senior-management-level individual responsible for responding to search warrants. This individual is responsible for ensuring that there is always someone present to contact legal counsel and to carry out the response procedures.

PROCEDURES

1. Outside counsel experienced in health law and federal enforcement will be on call as needed, with names and office/home/pager telephone numbers on file.

2. Designate someone to act as leader of the management response team at each company location who will receive the search warrant (or subpoenas)and, in consultation with legal counsel, will interact with the government agents.

3. Others should be designated to assist the company in monitoring any search, using a minimum number of people to reduce the level of confusion (include staff members who understand the company's electronic storage and communications systems). As part of their duties, they should reassure employees who will be somewhat distressed by the process and get them out of the way.

4. Reception staff members should be trained as to what they should do if government agents arrive unannounced, including:

    • To what office or room they should direct the agents

    • Who to notify to meet them (designated leader as noted above)

    • Possibly also a list of people who should be alerted

A predetermined call list should be in place, so that the names one the list can be alerted automatically concerning the search.

Anyone who is not part of the response team should get out of the way and should not try to interact with the agents. There is no obligation to give an interview during a search, but it is inadvisable to appear to instruct employees not to talk to agents. The best policy is to just let them do their job. Any questions by the agents should be directed to the designated lead person.

The lead person should meet the agents quickly and inquire politely as to how they may be assisted. He or she should take note of the agency represented by the agents and ask for the identity of the lead agent. He or she should make no attempt to copy investigators' credentials. To do so is a violation of federal law, and they will rightly object.

The lead person should request to view and photocopy the search warrant document. He or she should

carefully examine the search warrant (with legal counsel, if possible) to determine the following:

- The specific areas or locations it covers. He or she should attempt to work out an agreement to the degree possible of the areas of search as described in the warrant and maintaining reproduced copies of the records seized.

- He or she should ensure that the search is being executed during the hours indicated on the document (most warrants should limit the hours they can be executed, e.g. "daylight hours").

- Ensure that the warrant has not expired (all warrants should have an expiration date).

- Ensure that the warrant is signed by a judge (all warrants should be signed by a judge).

Send a copy of the warrant to legal counsel by the most expeditious means.

The lead person shaould also:

1. With legal counsel, if present), determine what specific premises the warrant covers and what specific documents/evidence investigators seek.

2. Point out any overt flaw in the warrant to the agents, and politely object to any searches outside the scope of the warrant.

3. Do not interfere if investigators go ahead and search in the objected area. Document the objection for legal counsel, and any results of the search may later be suppressed.

4. Request time prior to the search to consult with counsel to determine the appropriate course of conduct. It is likely that the request will not be honored.

5. Tell investigators if designated privileged files and documents are on the premises. If they seize any of these records, it should be noted that they had been advised.

6. Maintain a record of what happens, including number/identity of agents, areas searched, times of search, records/materials taken, etc. This is particularly important if patient records are taken, as they are not exempt from any search.

7. Allow agents entry into virtually anything within the defined location, including any room, locked cabinets, files, desk drawers, etc. This includes forcing entry. This may mean individual workspaces and personal privacy invasion. If a government agent(s) bearing a warrant does show up, bear in mind that they are acting as agents of the court. Any interference could well be viewed as obstruction of justice, an actionable offense.

8. Immediately contact legal counsel and the chief compliance officer, and provide details of the search warrant.

9. Request an "inventory list" of the documents and items seized by the agents. Ensure it is detailed enough to properly identify the documents and items taken by the agents. Maintain a separate record of the areas searched and documents/items seized.

10. Other than providing information to direct the agents to information requested, do not submit to any form of questioning or interviewing.

11. Always remain present while the agents are conducting the search.

Chapter 4 | Compliance program implementation planning

As part of this book, we want to introduce readers to a suggested compliance implementation plan. The purpose is to focus on implementation strategies in utilizing the templates and tools provided by this book. The best policy available to healthcare providers is a compliance program that complies both with the United States Sentencing Commission Guidelines for Organizations (Guidelines) as well as with the "Compliance Program Guidance" suggested by the Office of Inspector General (OIG). Compliance with the Guidelines not only prevents violations of the law, but it also acts in mitigation when violations of the law do occur. Conversely, failure to comply can have financial consequences and could prove fatal for a company.

The Guidelines were designed to create powerful new incentives for companies to implement effective compliance programs to prevent and detect violations of law and to induce self-reporting of violations. The OIG Compliance Program Guidance documents reinforce this message for the healthcare industry. These incentives are built into the formula used to calculate the fines and penalties.

Depending on the existence of an effective compliance program or absence thereof, the penalties may be significantly reduced or increased. The Guidelines promise no immunity from prosecution, but it is reasonable to expect that the existence of a bona fide compliance program would exert some favorable influence on prosecutorial discretion and willingness to seek reasonable accommodation and settlement.

Seven basic elements of a compliance program

The OIG believes that every effective compliance program must begin with a formal commitment by the organization's governing body to include all of the applicable elements identified by them.[1] Their guidance offers the same basic elements as the guidance provided by the Sentencing Commission, but it focuses these elements on the healthcare sector in general and Department of Health and Human Services (HHS) regulatory/legal issues in particular. As such, the OIG states that at a minimum, comprehensive compliance programs should include the following seven elements discussed earlier in this book (Chapter 2).

The most difficult part of compliance with the Guidelines is the need to document properly that a compliance program is a real and effective program. A written plan on the shelf is meaningless unless an organization can demonstrate effectiveness in the operation of the program.

The Department of Justice and OIG have taken a fairly hard line on providing real and convincing evidence that the program is effective in meeting the letter and intent of the Guidelines and Compliance Program Guidance documents. Although compliance with the Guidelines seems rather undefined, there are many steps a company can take to implement and provide evidence of a qualifying program.

The approach included in this book is designed to include these steps and is discussed below:

- Begin with an overall infrastructure to work in conjunction with other processes that currently exist within the organization. It will assist in the identification and resolution of a wide range of problems that could give rise to liabilities (e.g., fraud, kickbacks, conducting personal business on company time, sexual harassment, nepotism, billing and coding problems, wrongful discharge, fraudulent practices, OSHA violations, etc.).

- Focus on developing a program to assist employees in reporting such issues in a non-threatening manner, when they are identified.

- Ensure that the compliance program meets the general standards established by the OIG in the Compliance Program Guidance documents.

The methodology included in this manual illustrates how an organization can move to develop a compliance program that meets the criteria common to the Sentencing Commission and OIG *Compliance Program Guidance*.

It is difficult to outline a single approach to will fit every organization's needs, particularly where most have already begun to implement or have implemented a compliance program. However, the following outline will take a very generic, broad-based approach by using a four-step process to address all seven elements of an effective compliance program. It envisions moving on several fronts simultaneously. Therefore, most of the activities described in each step will overlap with successive steps.

Any organization may expect to receive the following tangible benefits from using the outline, approach, and templates:

- Reinforcement of corporate values and culture

- Proper infrastructure for the administration of the compliance program

- Better focus on compliance program goals

- Specific identification of potential compliance high-risk areas

- Heightened awareness of compliance issues

- Improved employee skills in dealing with these issues

- Enhanced involvement by executives/managers in promoting compliance

- Code of conduct relevant for management, employees, and government

- Reduced risk of "whistleblower" or "qui tam" actions by employees

- Facilitation of an effective auditing and monitoring program for high-risk areas

A four-step planning process for rapid compliance program development

Each of the four steps refer to relevant templates included in this book that can be adapted to almost any kind of organization or work environment. It is suggested that these steps be incorporated into the compliance planning process.

STEP I: Develop compliance program infrastructure

In Step I, it is suggested that that an organization focus on building a "top-down" structure for the compliance program beginning at the board of director's level and continuing through the chief executive officer/president, chief compliance officer, and other executives and senior managers. Specific activities in this step include developing:

- A board-level compliance committee policy document that describes the duties and responsibilities of the board in providing oversight of the compliance program development and implementation (Template 3).

- An executive compliance committee policy document that describes the duties and responsibilities of an executive-level committee in providing oversight of the compliance program development and implementation, differentiating the role from that of the board-level committee (Template 4).

- Compliance officer position-description policy addressing duties, as well as the attributes, skills and knowledge expected of a compliance officer. Preferably this would be developed and adopted before the compliance officer were selected or designated (Template 11).

- Compliance officer policy with specific procedures that will govern the operation of the function (Template 8).

- Compliance responsibilities of management (Template 5).

- Compliance as element of performance evaluation policy (Template 7).

This book will assist an organization in developing operating compliance policies and procedures that include the following written guidance/policies:

- Compliance records-management policy (Template 14)

- Compliance office confidentiality agreement (Template 12)

- Employee anonymity/confidentiality policy (Template 15)

- Non-retaliation policy (Template 19)

- Credentialing and sanctions screening policies (Template 32, 33)

STEP II: Develop standards of conduct

The code (or standards) of conduct is the written embodiment of the compliance program and the most tangible evidence of its quality. It is the first major foundation for a compliance program and represents a guiding set of principles for the operation of the company. The Federal Sentencing Guidelines call for effective due diligence and set forth certain steps that need to be taken, including the following:

- Use the code of conduct policy (Template 2) as a framework for code of conduct development

- Provide a written code of conduct, compliance policies, and/or guidelines or guidance on compliance behaviors

- Demonstrate the relevance of the code of conduct to the work environment

- Develop and disseminate the code of conduct to employees

- Ensure consistency of the code of conduct with policy and procedure manuals

- Ensure the code of conduct is understandable by all employees (10th-grade reading level)

- Integrate adherence to compliance policies and procedures into supervisor and manager performance reviews

- Reinforce the code of conduct through internal communication

- Train staff members on the code of conduct geared regarding application of policies to everyday situations

- Monitor and enforce the code of conduct through the compliance office

It is suggested that considerable effort be expended to involve a wide range of people in drafting the code of conduct. It will make for a more credible document and will make it easier to secure final approval from the executive leadership and the board of directors.

The first step in this process should be gaining approval for a code of conduct policy that outlines what the code of conduct should include and the expectations of employees regarding the application of the code of conduct. Gaining approval of such a policy document will pave the way for the actual drafting of the code of conduct. The executive compliance committee should be presented with the code of conduct for comment, suggestions, and approval prior to submission to the board of directors for final approval.

STEP III: Establish employee compliance hotline

A hotline provides a reporting mechanism through which employees can report criminal conduct or any type of wrongdoing by others in the organization without fear of retribution. It is recognized as an essential element of a compliance program intended to diminish culpability and gain mitigation under the Guidelines. The handling of calls through properly trained and managed hotline staffs have permitted interventions that could have otherwise resulted in litigation involving millions of dollars.

Hotlines can provide invaluable insight into management practices and operations. Callers use hotlines to report actual or perceived problems, thus providing a channel to identify issues warranting attention.

This book provides considerable guidance on the types of policy documents necessary for this element. It also addresses the issue of whether it makes more sense to operate the hotline in-house or to outsource it. In the vast majority of cases, the decision will be to outsource the answering of the calls. For making the decision on who to select for that function, this book offers suggested decision criteria that can be used. There are templates policies offered on how this function should operate within an organization:

- Hotline charter (Template 17)

- Employee compliance hotline policy (Template 18)

STEP IV: Communicating the compliance program to employees

It is important that the organization's principles, as defined in the code of conduct, be understood as an essential element of the organization's culture. It is equally important that the employees understand how the compliance program operates.

In Step IV, as with other steps, it should begin with deciding on just what the organization is willing to commit itself to in terms of compliance education and training, and then rendering that in the form of a compliance training and education policy document (Template 16). This policy should describe among other things:

- The types of training to which the organization will commit itself

- The frequency of the training

- The length of the training sessions

- The general course content

- The responsibilities associated with the development and delivery of the training

- The required documentation of training

Developing this kind of policy document should be done in advance of trying to develop a training program. To assist, this book provides a template that addresses most of these issues. It can then provide the framework for discussion and decision.

The training programs should communicate the expectations of employees in the workplace as described in the code of conduct and, in particular, address compliance high-risk areas and responsibilities. The programs should be delivered to all affected parties, certainly including employees and physicians.

A key element of any effective training program must be the visible commitment of executives, managers, and other supervisory personnel who are considered by the employees to be responsible for high standards of compliance-oriented behavior. Employees (including the compliance officer, compliance office staff, and organization executives) and board members should be trained. It is important to customize the training for each group to be relevant to specific roles within the organization.

Step IV activities may include:

- Developing a strategy to communicate the compliance program to employees

- Development of employee compliance training policy and procedures

- Compliance training roll-out plan

- Interactive training methodologies built on case studies

- Establishing a train-the-trainer program for employee and physician training

- Developing course material for the training sessions

Best-practice tip

Develop a work plan that addresses:
- Objectives for the seven compliance program elements
- Tasks to be completed
- Deliverables needed
- Time frames for completion

Following is a template for objective setting, defining tasks, and statements of deliverables for each task. This can be used as a starting point for a plan under development. Template 40 can be modified depending on what tasks and deliverables might already have been addressed. It is also located on the CD-ROM.

TEMPLATE 40

FOUR-STEP IMPLEMENTATION PLAN

	Objectives	Deliverables
STEP I **Develop a** **Compliance** **Program** **Infrastructure**	❑ Establish a Staff-Level Compliance Work Group to assist in Code development and/or revision. ❑ Establish Policies and program infrastructure. ❑ Identify proper support/resources for operation of the compliance program. ❑ Involve managers in understanding their compliance role/responsibility. ❑ Encourage employees to raise questions about conduct as well as the corporate standards of conduct.	❑ Work Group with legal counsel, HR, finance/audit, and operational areas involvement. ❑ Policy for Audit & Compliance Committee (TEMPLATE 3). ❑ Exec Compliance Committee Policy (TEMPLATE 4). ❑ Compliance Officer PD, Duties, etc. (TEMPLATE 11). ❑ Compliance Officer Policy (TEMPLATE 8). ❑ Other Compliance Policies (Templates 8, 9, 13 22 & 23).
STEP II **Develop Standards** **of Conduct**	❑ Provide simple, explicit guidelines for employees to follow. ❑ Ensure that all employees understand what is expected of them. ❑ Ensure that employees are putting standards into daily practice. ❑ Enhance corporate performance in basic business relationships. ❑ Ensure that business culture supports compliance conduct at all times. ❑ Build trust in the community that uses the organization's services. ❑ Provide a process for proper decision-making.	❑ Develop Code of Conduct Policy (TEMPLATE 2). ❑ Develop and gain approval for the Code of Conduct. ❑ Draft CEO cover letter for the Code of Conduct.

TEMPLATE 40:

FOUR-STEP IMPLEMENTATION PLAN (CONT.)

	Objectives	Deliverables
STEP III **Establish Employee/** **Compliance** **Hotline**	❑ Establish and publicize a reporting system through which employees and agents can report criminal conduct by others in the organization without fear of retribution. ❑ Create a reporting mechanism outside of the normal chain of command. ❑ Ensure the confidentiality of caller's identification and establish procedures to protect confidential information received on the hotline. Establish a mechanism to act upon information received from the hotline and, where appropriate, take corrective action.	❑ Develop Hotline Policies (TEMPLATES 17 & 18). ❑ Provide script for pre-recorded hotline message.
STEP IV **Employee** **Communication**	❑ Publicize and inform all employees of the adoption of the standards of conduct and the corporate compliance program. Ensure that key executives, the Board of Directors, and management publicly demonstrate their buy-in to the program as a part of this process. ❑ Develop and implement an initial education program for employees immediately after the company adopts the corporate compliance program, and document the company efforts to educate employees. ❑ Develop and implement a continuing education program using a group of in-house trainers. ❑ Document the training of all employees on the organization's code of conduct.	❑ Assist in the development of a master schedule for roll-out of employee compliance training. ❑ Develop Compliance Training and Education Policy (TEMPLATE 16). ❑ Develop and deliver 10–12 case scenarios drawn for training employees on how to apply the code. ❑ Develop Train-the-Trainer Manuals. ❑ Use training evaluation forms to measure and benchmark compliance training effectiveness.

TEMPLATE 41:

TIMELINES FOR IMPLEMENTION PLAN

DEVELOPMENT OF COMPLIANCE PROGRAM INFRASTRUCTURE

Workplan/Deliverables	Estimated Days to Completion
1. Organize staff-level work group for code development revision	14 days
2. Adoption of the Compliance Officer Policy Document by executive leadership/board	30 days
3. Adoption of the Board of Directors Committee Policy	45 days
4. Adoption of the Executive Compliance Committee (ECC) Policy by the board	45 days
5. Compliance Office Policies and Procedures	60 days

DEVELOPMENT OF CODE OF CONDUCT

Workplan/Deliverables	Estimated Days to Completion
1. Approval by the ECC and board of the Code Policy Document	30 days
2. Meeting with executives to define parameters of the code of conduct	30 days
3. Approval for mission/vision statements to be incorporated into the code	30 days
4. CEO cover letter to standards of conduct	45 days
5. Initial draft of statement of principles and code	60 days
6. Draft code circulated for comment	90 days
7. Presentation of code to ECC and board for approval and adoption	120 days
8. Disseminate code of conduct to employees	150 days

TEMPLATE 41:

TIMELINES FOR IMPLEMENTION PLAN (CONT.)

COMPLIANCE OFFICE AND HOTLINE

Workplan/Deliverables	Estimated Days to Completion
1. Adoption of Hotline Operation Policies	30 days
2. Selection of hotline vendor	30 days
3. Adoption of policies for investigations and resolution of issues	30 days

EMPLOYEE COMMUNICATION

Workplan/Deliverables	Estimated Days to Completion
1. Develop and gain approval for Compliance Education/ Training Policy	30 days
2. Training program plan and roll-out strategy	60 days
3. Develop 10–12 case studies drawn from the executive interviews for use in training	60 days
4. Develop and gain approval for compliance education/training programs	90 days
5. Develop in-house train-the-trainer training program with manuals and overview slides	120 days

The tables in Figure 4.2 outline suggested time frames for completion of the 21 tasks identified above. It is recognized that there are many variables that can affect these timelines. As such, it is anticipated that they will have to be adjusted considerably to match individual conditions.

Reference

1. See United States Sentencing Commission Guidelines, The Office of the Inspector General's Compliance Program Guidance for: Hospitals; Home Health Agencies; Clinical Laboratories; Pharmaceutical Manufacturers; Ambulance Suppliers; Individual and Small Group Physician Practices; Nursing Facilities; Medicare+Choice Organizations; Hospices; Durable Medical Equipment Prosthetics; Third-Party Medical Billing Companies.